MW00565209

Arteries in Harmony

Defending Our Arteries, Protecting Our Lives, and Preserving Our Happiness in the Era of Obesity and Diabetes

to Grant,

in gratitude!

Dr Anthony Pothoulakis

All rights reserved.

Copyright © 2018 by Anthony Pothoulakis

No part of this book may be reproduced or transmitted in any form or any means, electronic or mechanical, including photocopying, recording, or by any information storage or retrieval system, without permission in writing from the Publisher.

Copyright Notice

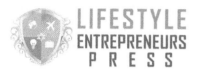

Publisher: Jesse Krieger

If you are interested in publishing through Lifestyle Entrepreneurs Press, write to Jesse@LifestyleEntrepreneursPress.com

Publications or foreign rights acquisitions of our catalog books.
Learn More: www.LifestyleEntrepreneursPress.com

Any unauthorized use, sharing, reproduction or distribution of these materials by any means, electronic, mechanical, or otherwise is strictly prohibited. No portion of these materials may be reproduced in any manner whatsoever, without the express written consent of the publisher.

ISBN 978-1-946697-99-8

My hope, my passion, is to help you.
The greatest compliment for me
would be if you all would allow me to have an impact
as you seek a better understanding of how to live a longer, healthier life.

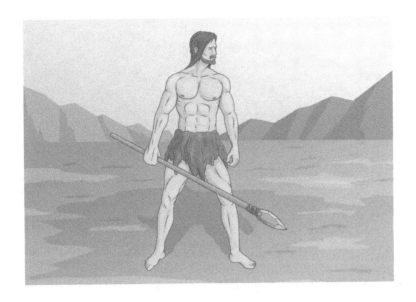

Dedication

I dedicate this book to the lasting memory of my father, Ioannis (Yiannis) Pothoulakis, an electrical engineer and an officer in the Greek Army corps of engineers. He was my first teacher in math, science, and reasoning. He is with me every day of my life. I also dedicate this book to my past and present patients who taught me so much about medicine and painted for me, in all its hues, the human nature and its language.

Acknowledgements

I want to thank my wife, Katerina, for the time she has given me functioning as a super-secretary for the entirety of this project and for the time she allowed me to steal from the two of us.

I want to thank the following individuals who helped me learn a thing or two from the immense domains of medicine and reasoning:

My professors George Daikos and Antonios Panayotopoulos.

My resident and fellowship directors and co-directors in Dayton and Toledo, Ohio and Birmingham, UK: Mr. SK Banerjee, Drs. H Verdain Barnes, Barrett Bolton, Howard Part, Hassan Mehbod, Richard Serbin, Partha Banerjee, Mohsen Sakhaii, Sylvan Weinberg, Donald Hammer, Agaram Suryaprasad, Satyendra Gupta, Theodore Fraker, Peter Temesy-Amos, Blair Grubb, Lucy Goodenday and Mark Burkett.

Our medical secretary, Ms. Maria Black.

The attending physicians that taught me so much: Drs. Roger Miller, M. Motekallem, Pierre Bamdad, Christopher Cooper, Tom Walsh, Ken Roush, James Bingle, Gopi Upamaka, Everett Bush, Carolyn and Charles Gbur, John Schwartz, John Letcher, Todd Monroe, CN Reddy and Ratnam Oza.

The physicians that offered me a job: Drs. Thomas Carmody, C. David Joffe, Miguel LaPuz, Scott Wolery, Elias Gavrilakis, Adel Shaheen and J.J. Shah.

My publisher Jesse Krieger, my dear friend Kristen Wise, our wise editor Zora Knauf and talented illustrator Stan Kurkula.

My co-author and invaluable partner in my first book *Abdobesity,* Mr. George Demosthenous

Foreword

One of the great transitions that occurred during 20th century and into the 21st century was the conquest of infectious disease by medical science. Up until that point acute infections were the leading causes of death and disability throughout the western world. The combination of both public health measures and antibiotics dramatically decreased the effect of acute illness and provided for a markedly prolonged life expectancy. At the same time modern science stabilized the food supply and helped produce an abundance of nutrition never before seen in human history. However as a consequence of these changes, chronic ailments such as hypertension, diabetes, and coronary artery disease began to increase in frequency and severity. At present these have become the major causes of death in the western world. By the end of the late 20th century in the early 21st century these chronic ailments have also begun to become the major causes of death in the developing world as well. Despite numerous efforts these illnesses continue to increase in both frequency and severity and have reached epidemic proportions.

In response to this Doctor Anthony Pothoulakis has provided a concise and thorough outline on the background, the causes, and potential solutions for these common and increasingly frequent health issues. While many have written on this subject for the public this book is unique in that it focuses on the important connection between diabetes and arterial disease. It provides a straightforward and easy-to-understand explanation of the causes of and the relationship between obesity, diabetes, and arterial vascular disease. It also provides a rational framework for dietary and lifestyle measures that could significantly impact the development and progression of obesity, atherosclerosis, and diabetes. The suggestions contained herein are practical and reasonably easy to institute and maintain. In short this book represents a welcome addition to the literature and a valuable guide to any individual whose goal is to be able to live a healthy and productive life.

Blair P. Grubb MD
Distinguished University Professor of Medicine and Pediatrics
The University of Toledo Medical Center
Toledo, Ohio
USA

Table of Contents

Why You Should Read This Book:

Death cannot be defeated, but health can be earned!

Obesity. Diabetes. Artery Disease. Problems big and deep. For all of us.

Diabetes, the most feared child of obesity, is so much more than simply high blood sugar, metformin pills, insulin injections, or controlling A1c. Diabetes brings complications that shatter the very foundations of our bodies. Treat diabetes with a casual attitude, give it 8–10 years, and it will literally eat you alive. And your family. And your community. And, in a generation or two, us all.

The plague of diabetes is hardly a US problem; China, Russia, and Brazil have as much diabetes as we do. While about 10 percent of US adults are diabetic, the rate in Mexico is 15 percent, and in Saudi Arabia one in four. One in four!

Obesity affects more than one in three adults in the US. Beyond contributing to diabetes, obesity is also responsible for high blood pressure, abnormal cholesterol, several forms of cancer, and knee arthritis and confers increased risk for atrial fibrillation, heart failure, and Alzheimer's, all prime killer diseases of our time.

As obesity and diabetes have spread worldwide, they are no longer simply an isolated epidemic; they are a global epidemic, a pandemic. Another pandemic, **artery disease** (high blood pressure, heart attacks, stroke, and sudden death) is a close relative and a frequent consequence of obesity and diabetes. And as 85% of diabetics die of artery disease, not high blood sugar, I refer to these conditions as a cluster, as the "obesity-diabetes-artery disease epidemic."

Obesity, diabetes, and their complications (including artery and heart disease) have high health, social, and monetary costs. They can be present for many years or even decades without symptoms or any kind of warning. They are all silent killers, as, when cholesterol plaques suddenly and unpredictably become unstable, these diseases can kill within a few minutes; the tragedy that the sudden cardiac death of a person in his or her forties, fifties, or sixties brings to those left behind is unimaginable. Obesity, diabetes, and their complications, thus, affect not only those who suffer directly from them but also their families, their workplaces, and our society. Looking at obesity and diabetes simply through the eyes of medicine misses the point. These diseases come at a monetary cost of almost one trillion USD per year and affect everything that lies at the intersection of money and health. They threaten not only lives but also family budgets (through insurance premiums, deductibles, and taxes), the entire health care system, and social safety nets like Medicare and Social Security. You must have heard those voices that warn us that Social Security and Medicare may not be around for the next generation. An anticipated increase in interest rates will only make the problem worse, as the government will be forced to pay more money to cover interest on its borrowing, with less money being available for Social Security and Medicare. If the fear of bankrupt Social Security and Medicare ever becomes a reality, obesity, diabetes, and artery disease will have all played leading roles. One can only imagine how our society would look and function without Social Security and Medicare! This dire prospect should define the vigor with which we should address the obesity-diabetes-artery disease epidemic today.

The obesity-diabetes-artery disease epidemic, on top of everything else, hurts our fight for a sustainable environment, as both livestock emissions (red meat being a favorite food choice for obese individuals) and the health and hospital care of diabetic patients significantly contribute to environmental pollution. So, every effort to curb the obesity-diabetes-artery disease epidemic also helps create a more sustainable environment and a viable and vibrant economy.

As obesity is caused by taking in more calories than we burn, the way to fight obesity must include:
- Taking in (through foods and drinks) fewer calories
- Burning (through movement and the development of body muscles) more calories

Taking in and burning calories is a lifestyle "choice"; in this respect, obesity (and its complications, including diabetes and artery disease) is a **lifestyle disease**. But since our lifestyle choices are, to a certain degree, determined by the social activities we must participate in, like going to school as kids and working as adults, obesity is also affected by **social factors**. No lasting solution to the obesity-diabetes-artery disease epidemic can be found without addressing both the individual responsibility for healthy lifestyle choices and the needed transformation of our social environment so that it supports rather than disrupts those healthy individual choices.

This book is based on my 30-plus years as a cardiologist and a practicing physician. My practice of medicine was based not only on cardiac procedures and heart pills but also on efforts to communicate science and impart knowledge, not just information, to my patients and their families. I found this communication necessary to bring us on more equal terms and make us stronger as we were trying to fight or prevent heart and artery disease. This book reflects my style of practicing medicine and my views on prevention and wellness, including the requirement that individuals accept responsibility for their lifestyle choices and whatever consequences these lead to. The book seeks to introduce, among others:

- The less familiar but more deadly face of diabetes, namely **diabetes as an artery disease**, leading to heart attacks, stroke, and sudden death
- Obesity and (type 2) diabetes as a **social problem**, not just a health issue
- An expanded version of **what a healthy lifestyle is**, going beyond just diet and exercise
- The fact that there are not enough hours in the day for the average working American to practice a healthy lifestyle
- My vision for implementing a **community-driven and community-wide, winning long-term strategy** against the obesity, diabetes, and artery disease epidemic by creating the **WellPals** (the friendly army of volunteers who will support healthy lifestyle decisions in the community and prime their friends and social contacts to become partners for wellness with their primary care providers),

by transforming school and the workplace, and by restricting dangerous foods and drinks

As an **engaged citizen and an active member of the society**, you have a stake in this issue, even if you are neither obese nor diabetic, even if you are slim and athletic, healthy and robust, and live in a place without hurricanes, forest wildfires, drought, famine, unstable economy, or social unrest. Getting to know better the many faces of the obesity-diabetes-artery disease epidemic along with its medical complications and its financial and social consequences will help protect not only your future health and the health of your loved ones but also the sustainability of our community and our economy, possibly for generations to come. It will make you a stronger person, a better spouse, parent, child, working adult, employer, or retiree, and a better citizen of our country and our increasingly globalized world. And, please, consider becoming a **WellPals** (see Chapter 7) and help in the fight against the epidemic.

My solution to the epidemic: living healthy 360 degrees

While the obesity-diabetes-artery disease epidemic seems to have the upper hand in most areas of the world, it is not unbeatable. A whole chapter in this book—Chapter 7—presents my vision, a cautiously optimistic vision for an all out war against the epidemic. I am deeply concerned that, so far, we have treated this aggressively spreading and destructive epidemic too softly. The solutions I propose, while based on the available scientific evidence and common sense, are not mainstream and should impart a paradigm shift in how we address the epidemic. As obesity, the foundation of the epidemic, rests on both lifestyle choices and conditions imposed by the social institutions of school and the workplace, we must address not only individual responsibility (for practicing a healthy lifestyle) but also a generous amount of social changes. The successful public campaign against tobacco smoking and the teaching of CPR to non-healthcare professionals can be used as guiding examples for an all out war against the epidemic. In particular, on top of fighting sugars and prolonged sitting at school and the workplace, the concept of **WellPals**, a friendly army of volunteers who will be knowledgeable enough to support public education and social transformation and help their social contacts seek medical care when they must, is also introduced in Chapter 7.

Arteries in Harmony

Obesity and diabetes kill primarily through artery disease: high blood pressure, heart attacks, stroke, and sudden death. And while very few people have perfectly healthy arteries, it is possible for most of us to pacify and stabilize whatever cholesterol plaques may be present in the walls of our arteries so that they never cause any trouble. This strategy of plaque stabilization (as opposed to the desirable but unrealistic strategy of zero cholesterol plaque) is achievable through prevention and wellness and by working closely with our primary care physician. **Plaque stabilization translates into prevention of heart attacks, stroke, and sudden death and is the essence of arteries in harmony**. It can be achieved through healthy lifestyle and, if needed, medical treatment of high blood pressure and LDL cholesterol.

Life is precious. Our bodies are precious. Our brains, hearts, livers, kidneys, and pancreases are precious. Arteries are double precious, as they support all our organs. As we cannot replace our critical organs or our bodies, we would like to preserve their health and, for the purpose of this book, keep our arteries in as good of shape and for as many years as possible—within the framework of aging, heredity, and the wear and tear that comes along with our daily responsibilities to our families, our jobs, and society.

Modern medicine, in spite of its almost miraculous advances, holds no easy fixes. Serious diseases, like artery disease, diabetes, emphysema, and arthritis, can be treated, but there are no magical pills or procedures to cure them. This is why prevention of a disease and its complications, if possible, is the smarter choice, both for you, as an individual, and for all of us, as a society. Through prevention we can use the natural and high-tech healing powers of our bodies to maximize wellness and preserve our health assets. In this way, prevention and wellness contribute to the health of the individuals and the robustness of our society. Abusing our bodies through a dangerously unhealthy lifestyle, day in and day out, and expecting that, when disease strikes, there will be a magical, inexpensive, and safe treatment—a miraculous pill—is plain wrong and utterly unrealistic. Choose wisely; invest in your health and wellness!

To your health,

Dr. Anthony
www.ArteriesInHarmony.com

Where Do I Come From?

For most of the 30-plus years of my medical career I have been a cardiologist. My duties have included invasive procedures in patients with heart attacks or chest pain, caring for acutely ill patients in hospital settings, seeing less ill patients in the office, and reading heart tests like ultrasound ("echocardiogram"), nuclear cardiology and other stress tests, and EKGs. My career enabled me to see a large number of patients and a large number of hearts, some healthy, some sick, and some very sick. One of my most dramatic experiences has been seeing the face of death in the form of a clot in a heart ("coronary") artery. As most of these patients were either diabetic or smokers, both preventable conditions, I became very interested in preventive medicine. I also became interested in explaining difficult and complex but useful health concepts to my patients and their family members. For this reason I also pursued studies in philosophy of science and mathematics, including approximate reasoning and fuzzy set theory. For the last 10 years, along with my other clinical duties, I have been active in the area of prevention. In 2012, I published *Abdobesity* my first book, with my co-author Mr. Demosthenous. *Abdobesity* showcased the direct role of abdominal obesity (belly fat) in causing the metabolic syndrome and artery disease, like heart attacks and stroke. I strongly believe that members of the public—not doctors or "healthcare" institutions—should lead prevention efforts if prevention is to be effective. So, in 2015, I started Arteries in Harmony, a company with the purpose of disseminating the principles of prevention and educating the public about the obesity-diabetes-artery disease epidemic in an easy to understand and actionable way. I have held a health blog ever since, and now I am publishing my second book, *Arteries in Harmony*.

My passion has been to provide a learning experience to those who care about the obesity-diabetes-artery disease epidemic by helping them understand how these killer diseases are connected to each other; that the "sudden" component in sudden death, heart attacks, and stroke may not be so sudden after all, as these diseases give subtle early warnings and can be prevented by following the right lifestyle; that these diseases threaten more than our health and the health of our loved ones, as they pose a threat to our progress, our economy, and the civil society. So, please, take advantage of my professional experience and what I have learned over my many years of studying and taking care of more than 100,000 patients face-to-face and become a credible source of advice to yourself, your loved ones, friends, and colleagues on issues related to the obesity-diabetes-artery disease epidemic.

How to Use This Book

Arteries in Harmony looks at the health, social, and financial effects of obesity and its complications, mainly (type 2) diabetes, high blood pressure, and artery disease, the top killers of our time.

Chapter 1 presents the obesity-diabetes-artery disease epidemic as a critical health, social, and economic problem that concerns all of us, not just those who are obese or diabetic. It points out that the fight against the epidemic can only be fought successfully by us, the people, through a community-driven and community-wide, long-term campaign. Scientific institutions, hospitals and doctors, pills, and procedures provide knowledge and help define the course and treatment of disease but cannot, by themselves, win the prevention and wellness game, as they cannot put "boots on the ground."

Chapter 2 takes on the biology of obesity, diabetes, and artery disease. It explains how fat cells strangle the key members of our metabolism and artery health:
- The liver, the main factory of our metabolism
- The pancreas beta cells, which produce insulin
- Our arteries and heart cells

It explains the connection between obesity, type 2 diabetes, high blood pressure, and abnormal cholesterol, all components of the metabolic syndrome. It also explains why most of these diseases are "silent killers," providing very few clues over the years before they destabilize our cholesterol plaques and suddenly clog our arteries.

In **Chapter 3** you'll learn ways to destroy your arteries, if you so wish. Key ingredients for artery destruction include not only a sedentary lifestyle and an unhealthy diet, but also smoking, stinting on your sleep, and abusing alcohol or drugs. Plus, you have to be patient, as youth will protect you for a couple of decades, even if you abuse your body.

Chapter 4 presents the exact opposite: the road to protecting your arteries and enjoying a long, productive, and healthy life. It is a mirror image of Chapter 3 and also compares two popular diets, the Paleo and Mediterranean diets.

Chapter 5 presents the difficulties and misconceptions that people are faced with as they try to change course, stop unhealthy habits, and start living healthier. These commendable people are actually the majority among us, as very few of us either have a perfect lifestyle or do not care at all about our health. In this chapter you will find practical tips as to how transition into a healthy lifestyle the best way possible.

Chapter 6 defines what a healthy lifestyle really is, going beyond diet, exercise, and not smoking. It incorporates elements like sleep, limiting sitting and very long work hours, treating high blood pressure or high LDL with medications, if necessary, getting age-appropriate screening tests and immunizations, avoiding alcohol and illicit drug abuse, avoiding long-term use of NSAIDs and opioids, having a rich social life, and avoiding falls and accidents.

Chapter 7 presents details of my vision for an all out war against the obesity-diabetes-artery disease epidemic:

- How to energize and mobilize the community through the creation of the WellPals, the friendly army of volunteers
- How to transform school and the workplace to include more moving and less sitting
- How to restrict the use of sugary foods and beverages

Chapter 8 is the Epilogue. Here you will look back through the journey of life, being active and productive into the third age, the challenge of Alzheimer's, and your legacy in the war against the epidemic.

Chapter 1

THE MAKING OF THE OBESE AND DIABETIC SOCIETY AND THE PEOPLE WHO WILL UNDO IT

"It's never too early or too late to work towards being the healthiest you."
—Unknown

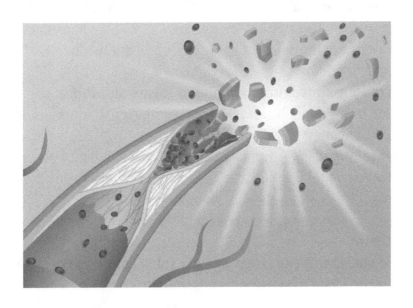

This is the age of obesity and diabetes. Why?

The facts:

While obesity in the US has been slowly but steadily rising since the turn of the 20th century, adult obesity has almost tripled over the last 50 years; more than two out of three adults are now obese or overweight. Similarly, type 2 diabetes has increased five times during the same time period, with about 1 in 10 adults being diabetic and 1 in 3 prediabetic! Childhood and adolescent obesity continue to soar.

The reasons:

- **Suburbia and the automobile**: people no longer walk to work or to the grocery store.
- **Screens of all kinds**: television, computers, and smartphones invite people to sit for hours on end, especially since screens are addictive (leisure) or necessary (work); for kids, screens usually win over going out to play.
- **Shifts in the US labor force:** there is 60% less physical activity required in the workplace compared to 50 years ago. Today a successful employee can be 100 percent productive and 100 percent sedentary.
- **Increasing consumption of added sugars and sodas:** energy intake from sweetened beverage consumption, for example, increased 135% between 1977 and 2001.
- **Living longer**: life expectancy in 1900 was 48 years versus 78 years now. As we age, we lose muscle, our metabolism slows down, and we gain weight (fat); also, our pancreas beta cells dwindle with aging, contributing to reduced production of insulin and (type 2) diabetes.
- The **successful campaign against tobacco**: not smoking increases appetite. However, smoking is much worse than obesity. Lung cancer, a deadly disease mostly due to smoking, has decreased by more than 30 percent in recent years as fewer people smoke, and it continues to decline by almost 2.5 percent every year.

What does the age of obesity and diabetes mean for our society?

Obesity and overweight are not only very common, they are also very serious as they are the driving force behind:

- High blood pressure (almost half of the adult population)
- Prediabetes (one in three US adults)
- Type 2 diabetes (one in ten)

Considering that diabetes and high blood pressure lead to heart attacks, strokes, kidney failure, and a host of other serious complications, these diseases result in a large number of people getting sick. The story does not end there: sick people can't work and need expensive medical care. Their family members suffer, as they have to take care of them. Their coworkers suffer, as they need to pick up the slack. The entire society suffers, as so many of these members lose their good health and so many others have to work around the ones who are directly affected by it and support them through their care, work, and taxes. In these (and many other) ways, the obesity-diabetes-artery disease epidemic is placing unprecedented stress not only on the individuals who suffer directly from these conditions but also on their families, their coworkers, the labor market, the tax base, the environment, and all of us—the entire society:

- The environment suffers when people consume animal fat, as livestock emissions create more greenhouse gas emissions than cars. How can we convince people to give up beef for fruits, vegetables, fish, and healthy fats?
- As people become obese, they develop high blood pressure, abnormal cholesterol, diabetes, and knee arthritis and get sick. Over time, they also suffer heart attacks and strokes and get even sicker. Sick people don't work. Who will work for them? Sick people need care. Who will care for them?
- Pancreatic beta cell function (i.e., production of insulin) declines as we age, even if we are not obese, making older people more likely to become diabetic. Diabetes leads to serious complications like kidney failure, heart attacks, and stroke. People with diabetes complications get sick, very sick. Sick people don't work. Who will work for them? Sick people need care. Who will care for them?

- Simply getting older makes us frail or makes us retire from our jobs. Most retirees (about 75 percent of them) don't work. With the baby boomers retiring, who will work in their place? Who will support them when they get sick? Who will pay for their Social Security benefits?

These questions emphasize the complex nature of the epidemic (health, social, and economic problems of immense proportions) and keep scientists, public health officials, and policymakers up at night, as what has been done up to now has failed to curb the epidemic; obesity rates skyrocketed since the early 1980s, and childhood obesity, in particular, has tripled since the 1970s and continues to be on the rise. Even the Speaker of the House Paul Ryan showed concern about the social safety nets in our society and said recently: "Baby boomers are retiring and we have fewer people following them in the workforce." He suggested that Americans need to have more babies or risk a collapse of entitlements like Medicare and Social Security. And while young families can work on the baby producing part of the equation, it benefits all of us to work on how to reduce the numbers of adults who become sick and unable to work because of obesity, diabetes, high blood pressure, artery disease, and their complications, like Alzheimer's, a signature disease of our aging population; diabetic patients are almost twice as likely to develop Alzheimer's compared to non-diabetics. And obese individuals, even if not diabetic, are at higher risk for developing dementia.

So what should we do at this juncture, when this epidemic threatens to destroy not only our health but also our civil society as we know it? On the one hand, the science about the epidemic is clear: added sugars and animal fats along with too much sitting and not enough body movement poison our metabolism, cause our muscles to shrink, make us diabetic, and increase our blood pressure and LDL cholesterol. Next stage is artery disease (heart attacks and strokes). It is as simple as this! On the other hand, simply understanding the problem hasn't made it easier to solve it. We do know that donuts, sodas, beef, and unlimited hours of sitting get us closer to obesity and diabetes, but we haven't been able to part with these things. Even scientists agree that what has been done so far to stop the epidemic has not been successful. As children are becoming obese at higher rates than ever before, what are we, as their parents, doing? As kids hold the future, what kind of a future are we helping them build? An obese and diabetic society? A large number of sick people who will depend on the few healthy ones for support? And what kind of action should we take now, before the specter of the obese and diabetic society becomes an irredeemable reality?

Advancements in technology and innovation have brought us comfort and progress (through washing machines, cars, computers, smartphones, and streaming), increased productivity (digital technology), and have improved our health (through clean water, sanitation, electricity, immunizations, new drugs and procedures to fight disease), but they have also made us addicted to screens and chairs and enabled our addiction to sugars and animal fats. While obesity rates have been gradually increasing in the US and the westernized world since the beginning of the 20th century, the world has never known as much obesity and diabetes as it exists today. Children get addicted to playing video games on the internet, talking to friends online, or watching YouTube videos; they no longer go outside to play. No wonder they get obese! And as children are our tomorrow, childhood obesity sets the foundation for an obese and diabetic society; obese children of today will become the diabetic adults of tomorrow, on their path to developing heart attacks, atrial fibrillation, heart failure, and stroke. So, it is high time we stopped being soft against the epidemic and advance to taking action. Here is what I propose we do:

- Identify what "progress" has brought to our everyday life that is, frequently, not real progress but, instead, is pushing us backwards, threatening to eliminate health gains of more than a century.
- Be determined and brave enough to change how we live, work, eat, and move, be determined to get outside our comfort zone (both as individuals and as society), and transform our workplace, school, home, and social environment to align "progress," "productivity," and "economic growth" with the health of the individuals and the sustainability of the community.

If the 20th century allowed the social and economic luxury of wasting the health and productivity potential of a large number of people, this century can't.

Are we doing enough?

As the unrelenting stress of the epidemic leaves its painful marks on us, both as individuals and as members of the community, it begs the question: are we doing enough?

- Are we doing enough for our children, who become obese in record numbers?
- Are we doing enough for our adults and retirees, one in two of whom has high blood pressure and one in three of whom is prediabetic?
- Are we doing the best we can to establish healthy conditions, at school, the workplace, and home to slow down the epidemic? In particular, have we engineered the workplace, school, and our homes to support our health as much as possible by keeping us physically active, eating and drinking healthy, getting adequate sleep, and limiting this unnatural and ever-present stress? ("stress eating" or "emotional eating" makes us eat unhealthy foods and is a key cause of obesity in our society. Are we doing enough to control it?)

There is need for immediate action to fight this epidemic. Who is going to fight it, where, and how?

Who should we entrust with the task and the responsibility of fighting obesity, diabetes, and their deadly complications? Who will be our soldiers and our generals? Science? Hospitals? Doctors and nurses? Public health officials? The Department of Health and Human Services? The government? The state?

Science has done its part; it has produced the necessary knowledge and given us the roadmap to fight the epidemic. Research is ongoing, and more relevant knowledge is expected to be available in the future. Science has made it clear that through inactivity and unhealthy diet we become obese and diabetic; and obesity and diabetes, along with smoking, inadequate sleep, and a host of other factors (see Chapter 6) cause artery disease, like heart attacks, stroke, and sudden death. An unhealthy lifestyle brings more than artery disease, though; it can cause a host of cancers, arthritis, and even Alzheimer's. Science has made specific and practical recommendations for nutrition and physical activity, for abstinence from smoking, and for avoidance of alcohol and drug abuse. Scientific organizations have an extensive internet presence with credible websites that provide comprehensive information. This is what you can expect from science. Science has done its part.

All of us American citizens deserve to be proud of our **preeminent scientific institutions** under the US Department of Health and Human Services (DHHS), like:

- **CDC** (Centers for Disease Control and Prevention. In its own words: "CDC works 24/7 to protect America from health, safety, and security threats, both foreign and in the U.S.").
- **NIH** (National Institutes of Health "the nation's medical research agency—making important discoveries that improve health and save lives").

These institutions lay out, through advanced research all over the world, what is the best we can do to keep our body healthy and well functioning for many years to come. They do define what is, in theory, wellness. They have websites where they explain in plain language what the problem is and what we need to do. But the actual practice of wellness is up to the individual and the necessary social transformations are up to the citizens; scientific organizations will not force you to adopt a healthy lifestyle or go to see your doctor when you need to.

One of the important contributions of the DHHS is providing crucial social safety nets like healthcare coverage through **Medicare** and **Medicaid** and promoting patient safety and healthcare quality in hospitals and clinics by healthcare providers (doctors, nurses, nurse practitioners, technologists, occupational therapists, medical assistants, nutritionists, and a host of allied health professionals). It supports "wellness efforts to prevent risky behaviors such as tobacco use and substance abuse and promote better nutrition and physical activity." The achievements of institutions like CDC and the NIH and agencies like Medicare and Medicaid are noble and significant. But as monumental and substantial as they are, they have not been enough to stop the epidemic:

- Childhood obesity continues to climb.

- Life expectancy for males in the US has been dropping for two consecutive years, something not seen since 1920s.
- Diabetes cases will continue to increase by as much as 1 million diabetics in the US every year and will do so, possibly, for decades.

According to one study: "The diabetes population and the related costs are expected to at least double in the next 25 years. Without significant changes in public or private strategies, this population and cost growth are expected to add a significant strain to an overburdened healthcare system." So, do not expect CDC, NIH, Medicare, or Medicaid, by themselves, to "wipe out" obesity and diabetes.

What about our high-tech hospitals and sophisticated medical procedures? Can they wipe out obesity, diabetes, and their artery complications? The short answer is "No." Obesity, diabetes, and, in large part, high blood pressure are lifestyle and social diseases and, as such, **will not be defeated without lifestyle and social adjustments**. Yes, there is bariatric (obesity) surgery that can help you lose weight and there is pancreas transplantation that can "cure" diabetes; neither of these procedures is a "slam dunk," however, and only a small percentage of obese or diabetic patients qualify for these procedures; only about one in a thousand diabetic patients receives a pancreas transplantation every year, and only one in 300 obese individuals receives a bariatric surgery, mostly gastric sleeve (where part of the stomach is removed). Moreover, these types of procedures change the patient's body and health forever. Pancreatic transplant recipients, for example, must take powerful immunosuppressant drugs for the rest of their lives so that their bodies don't reject the new pancreases; those drugs significantly lower the body's ability to fend off cancer or fight infections. No easy fixes exist! Bariatric surgery includes some less invasive forms, like gastric sleeve, where the change in the body's anatomy is relatively limited. However, even this less invasive gastric sleeve surgery has potential problems: it is not always effective in reducing body weight in the long run and can have several complications (e.g., perforation of the stomach or the esophagus, acid reflux, inflammation of the stomach or the esophagus, nausea, vomiting, difficulty swallowing, infections, bleeding, gallstones, spleen injury, or even death).

What about **hospitals, doctors, and nurses**? Hospitals, according to the World Health Organization "... are health care institutions that have an organized medical and other professional staff, and inpatient facilities, and deliver services 24 hours per day, 7 days per week. They offer a varying range of acute, convalescent, and terminal care using diagnostic and curative services." So, hospitals will be happy to treat diabetes and heart disease (for a price). But in the WHO description of hospitals and their mission, there is not a word about disease prevention.

Hospitals get their job done by using services from doctors, nurses, and a host of other "allied" healthcare professionals who operate high-tech devices to evaluate, diagnose, and treat symptoms and diseases. So, if there is an emergency—for example, you develop chest pain or slurred speech and you may think that you are having a heart attack or a stroke—what should you do? You should immediately call "911" and go to the hospital! There, highly trained doctors and allied professionals will use advanced technology and equipment to evaluate your symptoms, reach a diagnosis, and treat you accordingly. In cases of heart attacks or strokes, doctors and their assistants will try to open up the clogged artery and save your life. They will also prescribe medications to help protect your heart or brain from more heart attacks or strokes in the future.

Nurses work together with doctors to constantly evaluate how well you are doing, inform doctors about any change in your condition, give you prescribed medications, and help you in activities of daily living while you are at the hospital. Nurses frequently assist doctors during procedures. They will also explain your condition to you and your family and will prepare your transition from being a hospital patient to one who is discharged and able to function independently at home. Nurses are big on educating their patients; they will demonstrate to you how to use medications or devices at home and clarify what diet and other activities you are allowed to have till you fully recover; how quickly to expect your pain to subside, your function to return, your incisions to heal. Both doctors and nurses will advise you on a healthier lifestyle so that you can achieve what we call "secondary prevention." Secondary prevention is preventing a recurrence of a disease that has already happened, for example, preventing a second heart attack or a second stroke from happening again.

There is no doubt that modern hospitals and their personnel are extraordinary institutions that can truly save lives and improve your quality of living in case you are suffering from an emergency or a life-threatening condition. But don't expect to go in a hospital loaded with sickness and come out totally "fixed." In the case of heart attacks or strokes, for example, those cholesterol plaques that caused your heart attack or stroke may be present in many other places, all over your body and all over your arteries, a process that started in your teenage years. These cholesterol plaques continued to mature till you developed your illness. Don't expect those cholesterol plaques to be "flushed out" of your system and disappear by a miraculous treatment provided by your hospital or doctors. Yes, a stent will crush the plaque located in the area of the heart attack and create room in the artery for the blood to flow again; a bypass surgery will, literally, bypass those cholesterol plaques and create new paths for the blood to bring oxygen and life to your heart, but cholesterol plaques will remain untouched in most other locations in your arteries, in your heart, your brain, and elsewhere in your body. It is **your job**, through quitting smoking, taking appropriate medications, eating healthy, and practicing a healthy lifestyle, to help stabilize your cholesterol plaques and reduce the risk of a future heart attack or stroke. Prevention and wellness, through a healthy lifestyle (and control of high blood pressure or LDL with medications, if necessary) can either prevent those cholesterol plaques from forming in the first place or, if already formed, keep them stable, quiet, and harmless. Stable cholesterol plaques will be unlikely to cause a heart attack or a stroke and are more of a bystander condition than a deadly disease.

So, it must be clear by now that no doctor, no hospital, no pill, and no surgery or other procedure can, without serious side effects or other life-long consequences, cure obesity, diabetes, or any of their long-term complications. And while CDC, NIH, and our government do provide leadership, knowhow, and valuable, often life-saving services, they, by themselves, have not been able to stop obesity or diabetes. Let me repeat it: **hospitals and clinics,** by themselves, **cannot defeat the obesity-diabetes-artery disease epidemic**. The epidemic **will not be defeated by the discovery of a new pill or the medical innovation of a new procedure**. Only **wellness and healthy living,** as the result of healthy individual choices and brave social adjustments—to the extent it is possible and does not take us back to the dark ages or the Paleo era—**will hold back obesity and type 2 diabetes.**

Who else, then, is left to get the job done?

No one else but us, the people. Since the epidemic is caused, to a great degree, by a frequently practiced unhealthy lifestyle (inactivity from too much sitting and overeating too many sugars and unhealthy fats), the burden falls on our shoulders to get things straight, for ourselves, our families, our communities, and our country, every day of our lives. Can the job be done? Of course, it can, but it ain't easy. We are up against formidable temptations, strong instincts, and deeply rooted habits. Most of this book deals with the many obstacles but also the brave options and solutions that are necessary to defeat the epidemic. We are up against, for example:

- The temptations of tasty but dangerous foods and drinks and their powerful promotion by the food industry
- Our own instincts of craving sugars and animal fats and avoiding physical activity, if it is not necessary for our survival
- A tradition of centuries that considers the sitting position as the default one and, in many cases, an act of kindness ("please, take a seat")
- Deeply rooted beliefs that "hard work" is a good and noble thing, even if it deprives us of the very human need for sleep and even if it completely reverses our natural circadian (day-and-night) rhythm and makes us work the "graveyard shift," making us sick in the long run

So, how should we fight?

Fighting the obesity-diabetes-artery disease epidemic means fighting tooth and nail to prevent every stage of it. The epidemic starts with:

- **Inactivity** (too much sitting, too much screen time, not enough moving, not building up our muscles) and **unhealthy eating** (too many added sugars and unhealthy fats, not enough fiber); stinting on sleep, abusing alcohol, and violating other aspects of the healthy lifestyle (see chapters 3 through 6) can also play important roles.

- Unhealthy lifestyle then leads to **overweight or obesity** (especially abdominal obesity or belly fat).
- Being overweight or obese then **destroys our metabolism**, leading to type 2 diabetes, high blood pressure or abnormal cholesterol, (or any combination of the above, see metabolic syndrome;" see Chapter 2).
- An unhealthy metabolism then leads to **heart and artery disease** (heart attacks, stroke, atrial fibrillation, heart failure, sudden death).

The two fronts of the epidemic:

A. Individual level

Stage 1
As the "foundation" of the epidemic is obesity (or overweight) through inactivity and unhealthy eating, the first stage of our strategy is:
- **Avoiding inactivity**: no more than six hours of sitting a day, at least two-to-four hours of moving, complemented by light weights and stretching.
- **Avoiding unhealthy eating**: limit added sugars; choose diets like Mediterranean diet or Paleo (see Chapter 4).
- **Preventing overweight and obesity**, especially abdominal obesity or belly fat.
- Not smoking, getting adequate sleep, avoiding alcohol and drug abuse, and practicing the rest of the components of a healthy lifestyle (see Chapter 5).

Stage 2
If overweight or obese, we must fight to prevent diabetes (type 2), high blood pressure, and abnormal cholesterol, trying first through healthy lifestyle:
- **Increase our level of physical activities:** no more than six hours of sitting daily, at least two to four hours of moving, complemented by light weights and stretching (see Chapter 5).
- **Eat healthy**: limit added sugars; opt for Mediterranean or (modified) Paleo-type diets.

- While losing weight is a plus, you may be able to prevent diabetes, high blood pressure, and abnormal cholesterol through daily practice of a healthy lifestyle, even if you do not lose weight. Developing your muscles (without aiming at extreme muscle bulk like bodybuilders) will improve your metabolism, even if you remain overweight or obese.

If increased levels of physical activity and healthy eating cannot prevent type 2 diabetes, high blood pressure, or abnormal cholesterol, then you need help. You need to work closely with your family doctor or other primary health care provider. **Medications will probably be necessary** at this stage, in order to control diabetes, high blood pressure, or abnormal cholesterol and avoid artery and heart disease. For some obese people with type 2 diabetes, high blood pressure, or abnormal cholesterol, weight reduction (bariatric) surgery may be an option.

Stage 3
If you have already developed type 2 diabetes, high blood pressure, or abnormal cholesterol (especially very high LDL), then you need **both a healthy lifestyle and medications** in order to prevent heart attacks, stroke, atrial fibrillation, heart failure, or sudden death. You cannot do this alone; you need to work with your family doctor or other health care provider. A dietician is a must, but other medical specialists (for example, a diabetes specialist, an endocrinologist, or a cardiologist) may also be necessary at this stage.

Stage 4
If you have already developed heart or artery disease (a heart attack, stroke, atrial fibrillation, heart failure), then you need medical care from **a team of doctors** and other health care professionals, including your family doctor or other primary care provider, specialists (a cardiologist, a neurologist, a diabetes specialist), and a dietician. While **multiple medications** are usually needed at this stage, practicing a healthy lifestyle can still make a huge difference. Individuals at this stage may be limited in the kind of activities that they can comfortably or safely perform. They need to work closely with a physical therapist, an occupational therapist, or a personal trainer and choose appropriate, low impact exercises that their doctors approve,

with frequent breaks; every time they feel tired, out of breath, dizzy, or develop other symptoms.

B. Fighting the epidemic at the community level: a community-driven and community-wide campaign

We cannot fight the epidemic alone. Less than 3 percent of the individuals in the US consistently practice a perfectly healthy lifestyle and have achieved an ideal body weight. With less than 3 percent of the population doing the right thing and succeeding at it, it seems that the epidemic is almost invincible. How can we lead a perfectly healthy lifestyle when conditions around us force or tempt us to do the opposite? How can we be physically active when, both at school and the workplace, we are coerced into sitting, frequently in front of a computer screen? And how difficult is it to resist the temptation of eating and drinking tasty but dangerous foods and drinks that are not only inexpensive and available in abundance but also aggressively promoted?

Defeating the epidemic will require transformation of our schools, the workplace, the grocery stores, the restaurants, and our homes. And this is going to be tough. A special type of social activism, health activism, will be required. A certain proportion of the population need to be trained in the principles of cardiometabolic health, a curriculum not much different from what is presented in this book. If one considers that 18% of US adults are trained in CPR, one can see that it is feasible to train 2% of the US population to become **WellPals**, the friendly army of volunteers who will be among our social contacts and will:

- Support us at every stage of our fight against the epidemic.
- Help us flex our citizenry muscle to bring healthy lifestyle to our schools and the workplace.
- Explain—in detail—what a healthy lifestyle is and what the tricks are to achieve it.
- Prompt us to "know our numbers" (waist circumference, blood pressure, LDL cholesterol, A1c) and create our essential personal medical history.
- Persuade us to see our family doctor or primary care provider when we need to but may bitterly resist it.

- Help us create and maintain our own medical records; so that when we visit a doctor for the first time, the most crucial information is likely to be available. Consider that privacy laws like HIPAA have made the exchange of medical information between providers difficult. Also, hospitals are required to keep our medical records for only 5–10 years from the date of our last treatment, so some of the older records may be irretrievable and lost forever.

What kind of a return should we expect from investing in a healthier lifestyle?

Living longer by about 15 years, if the healthy lifestyle is practiced consistently. Even more importantly, we can expect less diabetes and Alzheimer's, less heart attacks and heart failure, less atrial fibrillation, and fewer strokes. We can expect better ability to function, enjoyment from life, even in our eighties, and minimized need for surgeries and other invasive procedures that can not only cause serious complications but will also render us unable to function for months at a time due to long recuperation periods.

Are there any knowledge gaps in the way people address the epidemic in their everyday lives?

Knowledge is power, and this is certainly true in the fight against the obesity-diabetes-artery disease epidemic. But it doesn't seem to be any shortage of information on the causes and potential solutions to the epidemic. So what are we missing?

- We miss a language that the "consumer" will understand without it being so simplistic that important elements of the epidemic are not communicated; the health information consumer is not a "patient" but a likely "patient candidate"; every obese, overweight individual with a diabetic parent and every prediabetic is a diabetic patient candidate. What is the right language to communicate this "knowledge," this probabilistic knowledge, to the vast number of diabetic candidates?
- We need to dispel the belief that diabetes is a high blood sugar condition; diabetes complications, and, in particular, artery disease (heart attacks and stroke) claim many more lives than high (or low, due to medication effects) blood sugar does.

- We need to dispel the belief that cholesterol plaques form only in the arteries of older people or that there is something magical and foolproof medically approved way to "flush" cholesterol plaques out once formed.

Other key messages for the informed 21st century consumer should include the adverse role of abdominal fat, the various paths that lead to diabetes, and the great value of keeping our arteries healthy.

The success of the tobacco campaign

In fighting the obesity-diabetes-artery disease epidemic, we do not need to reinvent the wheel. Think of our success against smoking and the many diseases, like lung cancer, artery disease, and emphysema, smoking is proven to cause. In the 1950s and 1960s, almost 50 percent of the US population were smokers; people used to smoke in public spaces, like work, restaurants, and airplanes, and advertising promoting smoking (even to minors) was ubiquitous. Now, only 18% of the US adults smoke cigarettes, smoking is prohibited in public spaces, and tobacco advertising is limited. There is so much we can learn from the spectacular public health success in the fight against tobacco. Why not start to treat added sugars, bad fats, and other practices that fuel the obesity-diabetes-artery disease epidemic in a way similar to tobacco products?

Excerpts from health institutions about the obesity-diabetes-artery disease epidemic

Here are a few excerpts of what big institutions are saying about the state of the obesity-diabetes-artery disease epidemic, its causes, and its effect on our society:

1. "As the prevalence and numbers of people with diabetes continue to rise—a result of changes in the way people eat, move and live, and an ageing global population—**the already large health and economic impacts of diabetes will grow.**"

World Health Organization, Global Report on Diabetes, 2016

2. "The number of Diabetes Mellitus (DM) cases continues to increase both in the United States and throughout the world. Due to the steady rise in the number of persons with DM, and possibly earlier onset of type 2 DM, there is growing concern about:

- The possibility of substantial increases in prevalence of diabetes-related complications in part due to the rise in rates of obesity
- The possibility that the increase in the number of persons with DM and the complexity of their care might **overwhelm existing health care systems**"

Office of Disease Prevention and Health Promotion, "Healthy People 2020," US Government

3. "By dragging down rates of productivity and siphoning off resources that could otherwise be invested in education, technology, social improvements, and private capital formation, obesity and diabetes hobble even robust economies, such as those of the U.S. and China. In poorer developing countries, their impact is even more manifestly immiserising. **Every nation thus has a competitive incentive to respond to these challenges in the interest of economic growth and the welfare of future generations.**"

Economic Consequences of the Obese, C. Ford Runge, Diabetes. 2007;56(11):2668-2672

4. "As one of the three most expensive man-made burdens, obesity continues to negatively affect the health of billions of individuals worldwide. The damage and costs associated with obesity consist of increased health care costs, decreased productivity, and premature deaths. As a preventable disease, reforms must be made to address obesity through education, fitness, media, and employers. **With rapidly growing obesity rates around the world, confronting the issue must be done soon rather than allowing the costs to become insurmountable.**"

The Economic Cost Of An Obese Society, Investopedia, April 17, 2015 by Trevir Nath

Responsibility

As we consider ways to confront the epidemic and wonder how we should best live our lives in order to stay healthy, and given what we know today about how lifestyles choices can affect our health and invite disease, I must emphasize the crucial role of personal responsibility. Notwithstanding the social conditions at school and the workplace that definitely contribute to too much sitting and unhealthy eating, we cannot simply go on pretending that symptoms we develop later in life as a result of our own unhealthy lifestyle choices are "somebody else's" fault and that someone else has to pay for them. So, please read and repeat the following sentences:

- If I have been smoking half a pack of cigarettes per day since I was 20 and I get emphysema at age 55, my shortness of breath is my fault.
- If I am a "no fruits or veggies" guy who has been enjoying donuts and candies on an almost daily basis, without being physically active, and end up with obesity and type 2 diabetes at the age of 60, my belly fat, my high blood sugar, and the need for insulin injections are my fault.
- If I have been diagnosed with high blood pressure since my thirties, refused to take my medications, indiscriminately used ibuprofen or other NSAIDs on a daily basis and against my doctor's advice (see Chapter 6), and end up in dialysis, my kidney failure is my fault.

Chapter 1 Questions:

1. How many US adults, according to the new definition of high blood pressure (December 2017, American Heart Association) have normal blood pressure?

2. Does bariatric (weight reduction) surgery hold the promise of defeating the obesity epidemic?

3. Mention some elements of modern lifestyle that are detrimental to our health.

4. As compared with those who smoke, eat unhealthy, and do not exercise, how many years longer can individuals who follow a healthy lifestyle expect to live?

5. Does obesity lead to high blood pressure, or is it the other way around?

6. Are most US adults who are trained to perform CPR health professionals?

7. Beyond negatively impacting people's health, what are some other effects of the obesity-diabetes-artery disease epidemic?

8. Can the use of smartphones make children obese?

Chapter 2

THE PATH OF MY BODY

*"If you do not take care of your body,
where are you going to live?"*
—Unknown

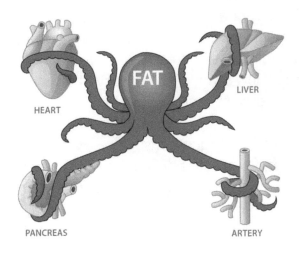

HEART

FAT

LIVER

PANCREAS

ARTERY

The obesity-diabetes-artery disease epidemic is a hallmark of our times. It is ours, and we own it 100 percent! It is caused when we don't take care of our bodies, primarily, through eating too many sugars and not moving enough, although heredity and aging also contribute. This epidemic is so big (two out of three adults in the US are either obese or overweight, one in two has high blood pressure, one in three is prediabetic, and one in ten is diabetic) that it is difficult not to stumble across someone with these conditions. The epidemic is also serious; its dark side is the many, and potentially life-threatening, complications of obesity and diabetes: the strokes, the heart attacks, the kidney failure, the heart failure, the blindness. The epidemic impacts not only on those who directly suffer from these conditions but also the community at large and the entire society and its institutions: the caregivers, the workplace, the family's healthcare budget, the society's safety nets, the taxpayers. As fighting the epidemic is a high priority both for the individuals who directly suffer and the society (which also suffers), all of us need to become familiar with its key aspects. So, whether obese, diabetic, a patient with artery disease, or thin, fit, and healthy, there are things we should all know about this epidemic. In this chapter will get to know some of the biology of obesity, type 2 diabetes, and artery disease, relevant to the epidemic.

Let's consider the following questions:
- Why do we face an obesity and type 2 diabetes epidemic today, throughout the world (a "pandemic"), as these conditions were not nearly as common 30, 50, 100, or a thousand years ago? (short answer: more calories in—mostly sugars, fewer calories burned—mostly sitting, and an unnaturally stressful life)
- How does obesity contribute to type 2 diabetes? (short answer: insulin resistance; longer answer: belly fat is choking the insulin-producing beta cells and makes liver inappropriately churn out more sugar when there is already plenty; sugars eaten and not burned end up becoming belly fat, feeding further into the vicious cycle: more unused sugar piling up in the bloodstream, more belly fat, less insulin production, more unused sugar piling up, and so on).
- Why do we consider **diabetes to be primarily an artery disease**? (short answer: most diabetics die of heart attacks of stroke—both artery diseases—not high blood sugar; diabetes makes our arteries

sensitive to cholesterol and prone to damage by cholesterol plaques).

- What else, besides obesity, makes us develop diabetes or suffer a heart attack or stroke? (short answer: heredity and aging makes us more prone to developing type 2 diabetes; smoking, diabetes, high blood pressure, high LDL, and chronic use of NSAIDs (see Chapter 6) contribute to heart attacks and strokes).

- What do we have to do to prevent obesity and diabetes or, if we have already developed them, how can we live well in spite of them? (short answer: know thyself, practice healthy lifestyle consistently, do not refuse medications if you develop high blood pressure, high LDL, or diabetes; work closely with your healthcare provider and ask questions).

Sugars, sitting, and stress

Cars, cell phones, computers, washing machines—all wonderful inventions that allow us to perform so many activities that we could have not even imagined 200 years ago: travel fast under safe and comfortable conditions; communicate with each other in real time and from the farthest places on earth; learn, work, and play at a stroke of a key, without leaving our home or office; go about our household chores with little effort (don't forget the 16th century that made chairs widely available). At the same time, all these wonderful artifacts have also hurt us; they removed the need for muscle work and body movement, a type of work that is not only a burden but also a condition for survival. Scientists estimate that the early man, before the agricultural revolution, was using his more than 600 muscles to lift objects, change posture, stretch, and move for about four hours a day, seven days a week. The life of the caveman, according to Dr Mark Walles, a chiropractor in England "... was an incredibly physically varied existence. We jumped. We ran. We pulled. We pushed. We relaxed. We climbed. We danced. We fought. *Homo sapiens* used to be a jack of all trades. Our bodies evolved to fulfil many roles."

How does this express the daily activities of you and me?

At the same time that we parted with our Paleo fitness, we made available an abundance of calorie-dense, sugary foods and beverages (not to mention excess fat and salt). "Humans crave high-energy foods, like fats and carbohydrates, because such food was hard to come by in the Stone Age, but can now be consumed in great abundance to the detriment of the body," says Harvard evolutionary biologist Jason Lieberman. Meanwhile, we consume only few natural foods like fruits, vegetables, tubers, roots, legumes and whole grains. We live a fast life; we opt for processed food or dining out instead of making our meals ourselves from fresh ingredients. We puff a cigarette, cigar, pipe, or hookah and drink several beers, glasses of wine, or servings of liquor. For at least some of us, this is a way to relax and escape stress.

Stress has been a permanent fixture in human history; however, the stressors of the cave man (and the few modern tribes of hunters and gatherers) were acute, severe, and pretty direct (being chased by a big animal or chasing one for food, finding shelter under unfavorable weather conditions, competing with other males for a female partner, defending yourself against an invader). Modern stress has more to do with unlimited wants in the face of scarce finances (when one may simply need a car, one may fantasize about a Lamborghini; a small shelter may not be as desirable as a mansion), facing deadlines, sometimes impossible demands for growth and productivity, sedentary conditions, and an unreasonable boss (or any combination of the above) at work and a spouse or kids (or parents) that bring their own unreasonable wants and demands to your face at home. This stress is:

- Chronic and lingering, never going away.
- Indirect and fuzzy rather than direct and precise (no one threatens your life; they may be simply threatening your income, your time, or your personal values).

This type of stress is unnatural and makes us:

- Eat more (usually unhealthy stuff like sugars or fast foods)
- Tend towards such a busy schedule that there is little time for exercise and personal time for relaxation or sleep
- Gravitate towards alcohol or drugs to "forget" our worries or smoke tobacco to help us relax

- Feel anxious or depressed
- Develop accident-prone behavior

Keep in mind that God did not make us to:
- Sit for 10-plus hours a day in front of a screen and call it "work"
- Eat 1,200-calorie cheeseburgers in one setting to satisfy our hunger
- Drink 160 calories in a glass to quench our thirst
- Inhale 7,000 toxic substances from the tobacco smoke of a single cigarette to pass time
- Abuse alcohol or drugs to relax or get high

When we abuse our high-tech bodies, this is the end result:
- A body that is obese and stripped of muscle and bone (tiny muscles and osteoporosis)
- A metabolism that is slow and poisoned (obesity and type 2 diabetes)
- Fat in places where it shouldn't be, like inside our belly or in between our liver, pancreas, heart, and muscle cells (type 2 diabetes, heart attacks, stroke, Alzheimer's)
- Cancer-provoking chemicals in our throat and lungs

These morbid and unnatural conditions not only cause untold human suffering but have also stigmatized our times and culminated in the current obesity-diabetes-artery disease epidemic.

All in all, obesity and diabetes kill mainly because of artery disease; 85% of diabetics die not of high blood sugar but of heart attacks or stroke—both artery diseases. And while, on the surface, the treatment of diabetes emphasizes pills or insulin to control the high blood sugar, the real battle is fought on another front, the insides of our arteries. The one who manages to keep his arteries as free of blockages and clots as possible and fend off heart attacks, stroke, or leg gangrene is the one who has really triumphed over diabetes, avoiding its deadliest complications. Here is why:
- Heart attacks start as disease in the arteries that feed the heart, called "coronary arteries."
- Most strokes happen because of clots in the brain arteries or inside the heart itself (this is the case in atrial fibrillation-related stroke).

Understanding arteries and artery disease, how it starts, and how it evolves over time is a major theme in this book. Our arteries are our lifelines: critical, essential, but at the same time, so vulnerable!

Arteries and artery disease

Our arteries are highly sophisticated tubes that form a complex network of highways, avenues, roads, and alleys that helps transport life-giving blood from the heart to every cell in the body, no matter how remote. Blood carries nutrients, oxygen, and a variety of cells that provide the body with the goods and services it needs. By serving all body organs, arteries are indispensable; no organ can survive without the constant flow of life and nutrients that arteries bring. This is why artery disease, like heart attacks and stroke, can have such catastrophic consequences: you block blood flowing down a heart artery, you cause a heart attack; you block blood flowing down a brain artery, you cause a stroke. As the arteries are hard at work 24/7, they are subjected to tremendous wear and tear and thus, are very vulnerable, making artery disease as common as it unfortunately is (number one killer disease in the US).

Do you know when and how heart attacks and stroke start? Artery damage does not happen overnight. What starts artery damage is fat inside our arteries. Fat in food or cholesterol produced by our liver (mostly due to heredity, not diet) enters the bloodstream and can damage our arteries as cholesterol starts being deposited in the artery wall. This initial stage of cholesterol plaque is already underway by late childhood. The first visible sign of cholesterol artery disease is called **fatty streaks** (small and inconspicuous lines of fat in the artery wall). It is the only stage of artery disease that is reversible. From there onwards, artery disease develops slowly but inexorably and **mature cholesterol plaques can be "appeased" but cannot be reversed**. In simple terms, **once you develop cholesterol plaques, they will never go away.** It is important to know, however, that **if those plaques remain stable, they will not threaten your life or your health.**

The final blow in a heart attack or a stroke comes suddenly and quickly in the form of a clot. Blood clotting is a natural, life-saving mechanism that allows arteries to rapidly stop bleeding when injured. As prolonged and severe bleeding can kill us, it takes only one to four minutes for a clot to form and plug the artery wound, stopping the bleeding. Imagine how many million lives must have been saved this way, especially at the time of our ancestors, when injuries were common and there were no emergency departments or trauma surgeons. In cholesterol artery disease, however, the reason for the clot formation is not bleeding but a sudden and unpredictable instability of a mature cholesterol plaque in the wall of that artery. A cholesterol plaque that has matured over decades hides in its depths chemicals ingredients similar to the ones present in an externally injured artery. In this way, the flowing blood is fooled into thinking we are bleeding and rushes to form a clot to plug the hole. In the case of an unstable cholesterol plaque, though, the clot formation (which still takes only one-to-four minutes to form) is not life-saving; it is deadly! If this clotted artery is one that feeds the heart or the brain, what follows is a heart attack, a stroke, or sudden death.

What is important to remember is that: while we start life endowed with healthy arteries and healthy hearts, over the course of a few decades, cholesterol plaques may develop all over our artery network and can then become suddenly and unpredictably unstable, resulting in heart attacks, stroke, or sudden death.

What other factors, beyond diabetes, obesity, aging, and heredity can also damage and destroy our arteries?
- Smoking
- High blood pressure
- Abnormal cholesterol (high LDL, elevated triglycerides, or low HDL)
- Unhealthy eating
- Lack of daily exercise
- Drinking more than moderate amounts of alcohol
- Not getting enough sleep, at least seven hours a night
- Chronic use of certain medications, such as NSAIDs, like ibuprofen or naproxen (see also Chapter 5), and opioids like morphine.

Thus, taking good care of our arteries from the get go (as early as childhood) is essential for our survival and well being. There is also good scientific data that shows that what works well for our arteries can also prevent cancer, emphysema, Alzheimer's, and even depression (see Chapter 6). Thus, it is not an exaggeration to state that **wellness and prevention start with keeping our arteries healthy.**

Common forms of artery disease:

- Coronary artery disease: blockages and cholesterol plaques in the arteries that feed the heart
- Cerebrovascular or Carotid artery disease: blockages in the arteries that feed the brain
- Peripheral vascular disease: blockages in any arteries other than coronary arteries, especially the arteries that feed our legs

High blood pressure ("hypertension," see below) is also a form of artery disease.

If our arteries were as visible as our skin is, we would be so scared and concerned with what we saw that we would definitely embrace healthy living and any other intervention that can protect our arteries. Now, in order to talk intelligently about obesity, diabetes, and artery disease, we need to talk about a number of different areas in the body. Let's get started.

Cells

The cell is not only the unit of life; it is also the unit of disease. In this way, getting to know what a cell is helps us understand both health and disease. So, let's take a brief look at the amazing world of cells and organs that make up our body. These few interesting bits of information can help us better understand the biology of obesity, diabetes, and artery disease.

Our bodies consist of about 37 trillion cells. There are over 200 different types of cells, each endowed with highly sophisticated parts and uniquely specialized to perform distinct functions. Did you know, for example, that each one of our cells has many more sensors and control systems than a high-tech modern car that is 3,000 quadrillion times bigger? A Lamborghini or a Ferrari does not have half the sophistication and complexity of a single liver or pancreas beta cell!

The following are examples of the variety of human cells and their diverse functions:

- Liver cells are chemical wizards and are among the most industrious of human cells; they absorb and process carbs, fat, and protein; they produce glucose (sugar) and cholesterol from scratch, along with blood clotting and fat-shuttling proteins; they store vitamins and minerals; they filter blood; they detoxify alcohol and medications and secrete bile that aids in fat digestion. Liver cells can also regenerate.
- Pancreas cells produce insulin, one of the most important hormones, that regulates the metabolism of carbs, fat, and protein. They also produce digestive enzymes. Pancreas cells do not regenerate.
- Muscle cells contain proteins that slide against each other, resulting in motion.
- Fat cells absorb, process, and store fats and secrete hormones and inflammatory chemicals.
- Nerve cells process and transmit information in the form of electrical and chemical signals.
- All cells are in continuous flux and can change as quickly as 500 times in a second! Thus, **one second is a long time** on the time scale of our biology, whether in health, aging, or disease.

Now that you know a little more about cells, we need to talk about metabolism.

Metabolism

We have all heard the term metabolism, but what is it, and how does it actually affect our weight and health? Our body is in a continuous flux, changing all the time. For this reason, our body is expensive to run. Every single day we destroy and recycle about 2% of our cells and their chemicals! This high turnover is achieved through billions of chemical reactions. All these reactions that are necessary for our body to stay alive and function well make up what scientists call "metabolism."

The pancreas and the liver essentially define a large part of our metabolism (not counting the brain, who is the "master" of all our organs). Located deep in our belly and behind the stomach, the pancreas is most important for the production of **insulin**. Insulin is more than just a blood sugar hormone controlling carb metabolism. Insulin also regulates the metabolism of fat and protein. Insulin spikes after we eat carbs and helps get sugar inside the cells to be used as fuel. Insulin also signals the liver that there is an abundance of sugar in the bloodstream.

The liver is the central metabolic factory and a major detox center of our bodies. All digested and absorbed food is channeled through the portal vein (a one-way highway that leads from the stomach and gut to the liver) and must clear the liver before entering the bloodstream. The belly fat of an obese individual attacks the liver through the portal vein, making it a **"fatty" liver**. This "fatty" liver behaves in a very abnormal way as it:

- No longer listens to insulin but, instead, keeps producing sugar from scratch, even when there is an abundance of it in the bloodstream. This condition is called **"insulin resistance"** and is a prelude to the development of type 2 diabetes.
- Produces bad chemicals that promote the development and destabilization of cholesterol plaques in our arteries, setting the stage, over time, for heart attacks and strokes.

According to the American Liver Foundation, fatty liver affects up to 25% of people in the United States.

Now you know that the pancreas and liver control metabolism, but diet is a factor as well. How do obesity-reducing diets affect our metabolism? When overweight, it is tempting to follow strict diets in an attempt to lose weight. However, keep in mind that when we reduce the amount of food ingested, our metabolism slows down as the body tries to conserve energy. Our ability to function is affected and we become moody. We cannot fend off infections as well as before. We also start burning muscle to use for energy; losing muscle slows down our metabolism even further, leading to a vicious cycle. Thus, do not fall easily for diets that reduce calories excessively without consulting your physician. At the other diet extreme, when we follow an unhealthy diet and take in more calories than we burn, we gain weight as those extra calories become fat. Once the normal fat stores under the skin are filled to capacity, we start storing fat in the belly. This **belly fat is an abnormal and dangerous condition**. As we mentioned earlier, belly fat is directly connected to the liver through the portal vein. In this way, belly fat becomes fatty liver and fatty liver becomes an agent of artery disease.

So, what should we strive for, in an attempt to maintain a healthy weight and keep our metabolic rate high?

- Control the total amount of calories you consume, first by cutting out unnecessary food items, like the worst carbs (cookies, desserts, baked goods, sugary beverages) and the worst fats (cold cuts, animal fat, fast foods).
- Consume adequate quantities of the good carbs (fruits, vegetables, whole grains), good fats (olive and canola oil, fish, avocado, dark chocolate, and unsalted nuts), and lean protein (skinless poultry, low-fat dairy, legumes, seeds).
- Increase the level of your physical activities to include two to three hours a day of moderate intensity aerobic exercise (walking, swimming, using a treadmill desk or standing desk, or just moving around) and, additionally, perform moderate intensity strengthening exercises (weights, resistance bands, push ups, sit ups, and squats), and stretching.
- Use physical activities that involve strengthening, stretching, and balance exercises to not only burn calories but also build muscle and protect your joints and bones by avoiding injuries and falls.
- Resist the temptation to pick up smoking because of its appetite-suppression effects. Smoking can hurt your health worse than obesity can.

Does our diet really make a big difference in our health? Short answer: *YES!*

Using the right mix of good carbs, good fats, and lean proteins:

- Keeps you full and satisfied without making you gain weight
- Gives your body the nutrients it needs (protein, water, antioxidants, fiber, and energy)
- Keeps your arteries healthy
- Cuts significantly your risk for developing cancer

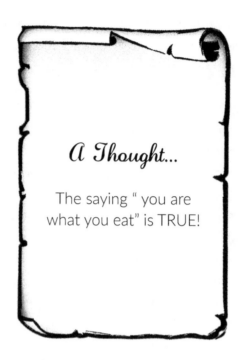

A Thought...

The saying " you are
what you eat" is TRUE!

Say your diet consists mostly of junk food, but you manage to stay thin. So,
what's the problem?

Junk food contains too many calories, too much salt, too much bad (animal)
fat, and too much sugar. Since you are thin, the amount of calories may not
be a problem. However, the amount of salt, sugar, and fat still is.

- Too much salt can increase your blood pressure. It is worse when
  you are both obese and you consume too much salt, but even slim
  individuals will experience higher blood pressure, especially after
  the age of 30 and when there are hereditary factors at work.
- Too much sugar will challenge your pancreas, even if you maintain
  a healthy weight. The pancreas needs to produce as much insulin
  as needed in order to shuttle the blood sugar inside the cells to be
  used as fuel. Thus, every time we ingest sugary foods or drinks, our
  beta cells squeeze as much insulin as is needed to put sugar inside
  the cells. The more refined the sugars, the more insulin and the
  faster needs to be produced. Repeat this exercise multiple times
  a day over a course of a few decades, add an element of heredity,
  and you see type 2 diabetes coming.

- Too much bad fat is likely to raise our triglycerides and bad cholesterol (LDL), even if we are thin. High LDL, in particular, means more widespread and more unstable cholesterol plaques in our arteries (those plaques will never melt away); that is the real trouble.

So, are you taking good care of this high-tech body of yours? If you had a Lamborghini, wouldn't you be putting the highest-octane gasoline available to keep its engine cylinders in as a pristine condition as possible? As your body is infinitely more complex and high-tech but even more vulnerable than a Lamborghini—and you are stuck with only one body for the rest of your life—it deserves the purest nutrients (water, good carbs, good fats, and lean protein) that will keep its arteries in as a pristine condition as possible. So "drive" your body every day the way you would drive a Lamborghini!

Did you know that our body is made up of:
- Water (about 50 percent of our body weight).
- Muscles (about 50 percent of the body weight in a young, fit man and 35–40 percent in a young, fit woman).
- Fat (20–25 percent of body weight in healthy, non-obese men and 25–30 percent in healthy, non-obese women).
- Almost 99 percent of the human body is made up of six elements: oxygen, carbon, hydrogen, nitrogen, calcium, and phosphorus.
- Sodium, although it makes up only one thousandth of the body, plays a key role in the development of high blood pressure.

Also, consider that whereas most of our organs can also use fat as a fuel, the brain cannot and depends on a constant supply of sugar. Brain cells can use sugar without the need for insulin.

If you are of a younger generation, you may not know this, but listen closely: the muscle content of our body declines with age and sedentary lifestyle, and the older you get, the harder it is to produce new muscle, in spite of exercise and adequate protein intake. So, take good care of your muscles by using them frequently, day in and day out, while avoiding injuries.

Sugars: simple and mean or complex and nice

Sugars are very important components of our diet. Sugars are either simple (small and quickly absorbed through the stomach and the gut) or complex (starchy and slowly absorbed). Simple sugars are found in table sugar, sugary beverages, refined grains, cookies, candy, desserts, milk, and fruits. Starchy sugars are found in green vegetables, whole grains, brown rice, potatoes, sweet potatoes, corn, peas, beans, lentils, quinoa, and couscous. Foods rich in complex carbohydrates are usually good sources of important nutrients (other than sugar), like vitamins, minerals, and fiber. Out of simple sugars it is mainly fruits and milk that are good for our health, as sugar in whole fruits (fructose) is combined with fiber and milk sugar (lactose) is combined with protein. The remainder of simple sugars in foods like candies, desserts, donuts, and other baked goods made out of refined grains, white bread, white pasta, white rice, sugary beverages, and cookies are bad for our health for the following reasons:

- They are "empty calories," as, beyond energy, they have nothing else to offer (no fiber, no vitamins, no minerals, no protein).
- Being easily absorbed after eaten, they lead to spikes in blood sugar that stress the pancreas beta cells, forcing them to release insulin quickly. These insulin spikes, beyond stressing the valuable pancreas beta cells, also cause a mild hypoglycemia and hunger pangs within the next two hours that force us to eat again and again and again!

Unlike simple sugars, complex sugars and sugar in milk and fruits provide not only energy but also other important nutrients (fiber, minerals and vitamins, and, in the case of milk, protein). Their gradual absorption into the bloodstream treats the pancreas beta cells more gently and insulin spikes are avoided. These good carbs keep us full for several hours so we are not forced to eat often. For all these reasons, the National Institutes of Health suggests eating more complex carbohydrates and limiting simple sugars from candy and sweets, which have little or no nutritional value. The American Heart Association recommends limiting simple sugars (not counting sugars in milk or fruits) to no more than 25 to 40 gm of sugar daily. Unfortunately, simple sugars abound in modern diets, in great part due to their longer shelf lives (good for business) and the instant and strong pleasure associated with their consumption. Eating too many simple sugars is one of the main causes of obesity, diabetes, and artery and heart disease. In spite of simple sugars being dangerous, they are treated with a cozy attitude, frequently regarded as "comfort food."

Fat

We all have some fat, but when it gets to be too much it can be dangerous. Fat, especially inside our bellies, is the essence of obesity and a key ingredient of the metabolic syndrome type 2 diabetes and artery disease. Fat is also the venue of choice for energy storage, as it can hold more than twice as many calories compared to carbs or proteins.

About 20–25 percent of the body weight in healthy men and 25–30 percent in healthy women is fat under the skin. If, instead of fat, protein or carbs were the way our body stored energy, we would weigh 40–60 pounds more! Imagine the added strain on our joints, hearts, and lungs under such conditions!

The normal site of fat residence is under the skin. Fat under the skin is not only normal; it is necessary. Let me say that again: **"Fat under the skin is not only normal; it is necessary!"** If you have some arm fat and leg fat, that is okay. This "subcutaneous" fat is the normal way of storing energy in our body; it also functions as an insulator and helps keep body temperature stable; additionally, subcutaneous fat protects muscles and bones from injury.

However, **NOT ALL FAT IS CREATED EQUAL!** While subcutaneous fat (fat under the skin) is normal, belly fat is NOT. Once the capacity to store fat in its normal place under the skin is exceeded, we start storing fat in other places, like inside our belly and between our body organs and muscle. If you do have belly fat, it is fair to assume that you also have fat abnormally present inside and around your liver, pancreas, heart, muscles, and arteries. Presence of fat in these locations is a dangerous condition and an agent of destruction and disease. All in all, the only natural place for fat is under the skin. As we gain weight beyond what is normal, fat expands to other body areas. Practically, fat keeps bad company to any (other than the skin) body organ.

Question: When there is fat inside our belly, where else is fat hiding?
Answer: Fat is also hiding inside our:

- Heart
- Liver
- Pancreas
- Muscles

Fat is also hiding around our arteries. And all these hideouts are a sign that both our metabolism and our heart and arteries are on the path to destruction.

- Here is how abnormal fat damages its host:
- In the liver ("fatty liver"), it creates **insulin resistance** that contributes to high blood pressure and abnormal cholesterol, eventually leading to artery disease, like heart attacks and stroke.
- In the pancreas, it **directly damages the beta cells** that produce insulin and contributes to type 2 diabetes.
- Inside and in between our heart cells, fat makes the **heart muscle stiffer**, unable to relax normally and accommodate the oxygen-carrying blood coming from the lungs. This is a very common condition, especially after the age of 40. It is called "**diastolic dysfunction**" and can make us short of breath when physically active. At a more advanced stage, fat in between the heart cells makes the heart weaker; it can also cause a common and serious abnormal heart rhythm called "**atrial fibrillation**," a stroke-prone condition.
- Inside and around muscle, fat contributes to insulin resistance, makes muscles weaker, and slows down our metabolisms.
- Around the arteries, fat contributes to widespread cholesterol plaque in the artery wall ("**atherosclerosis**").

Are fat cells only for fat storage? No. They also produce and secrete a host of hormones and other chemical signals that, in health, help to regulate metabolism and energy storage. However, as the body fat stores expand in obesity, these fat-derived chemicals contribute to insulin resistance and establish a damaging proinflammatory state throughout our bodies (you must have heard that too much inflammation is not good for your health). **Belly fat is a serious warning that disease is already happening inside**

you. Be grateful that, thanks to our tremendous body reserves and healing power, this disease process has not yet bore the fruits of evil and, please, do something to stop it; for the sake of yourself, your loved ones, and our society.

Muscle

As muscle makes up almost half of our body weight, it plays a huge role in burning calories and determining the rate of our metabolism; a muscular body has a faster metabolism than a body without well-developed muscles. When we use our muscles, sugar moves into the cells without the need for insulin. In this way, a muscular body can fight insulin resistance and cancel out many of the ill metabolic effects of belly fat. Did you know that muscle burns calories even when we are asleep? The importance of muscle is such that the American Diabetes Association recommends at least 10–15 minutes every other day of light or moderate weight lifting and other resistance exercises for all diabetics. If resistance exercises work for diabetics, they work even better for the prevention of diabetes! So, when you try to lose weight in order to become healthier or prevent diabetes, don't forget building muscle, as muscle is necessary for the health of our metabolism and prevention of type 2 diabetes.

There is a difference, though, between lean muscle and excessive, bulk muscle developed through heavy weight lifting! Heavy weight lifting can cause straining ("isometric exercise") and is dangerous for our health, as during straining, blood pressure can rise to extremely high levels. These damaging high blood pressure levels can be sustained for up to 20 minutes after we are done lifting weights, causing, over time, strain to both the heart and the aorta (the main artery of the body). This may result in an abnormally thick heart muscle (hypertrophy of the heart, not a good thing) and aneurysms in the chest ("thoracic aortic aneurysms").

On the other hand, moderate weight lifting helps build muscle without causing dangerous blood pressure elevations. Thus, plan to always complement aerobic exercise ("cardio") with some strengthening exercises. Your muscles are the supermen of your metabolism; don't let them wither!

And remember that muscle and joints are strong allies; if our joints are not healthy, muscle use results in pain!

Joints

Healthy joints support our muscles so that bones don't rub against each other and our muscles can move smoothly. In this way, healthy joints help us use our muscles, burn calories, and maintain a healthy metabolism. Painful joints, on the other hand, not only prevent us from using our muscles due to hurting, they also force us to use painkillers. This can be dangerous for our health, as some of the most effective painkillers, like ibuprofen or naproxen (NSAIDs, see also Chapter 5), if taken daily for months or years, can cause heart attacks and kidney failure.

The sad reality is that cartilage, the shock absorber of our joints, once damaged, has a limited capacity to regenerate and practically stops forming very early in life. A study by Katja M. Heinemeier et al. published in July of 2016 in the journal *Science of Translational Medicine* found that cartilage collagen stops regenerating when we stop growing during our teenage years. While there is active research in cartilage regeneration, we are currently unable to produce cartilage that functions as well as the original cartilage we have in the joints as adolescents or young adults. So, **protect your joints to be able to use your muscles!**

Here is how healthy joints contribute to our artery health and help us fight against the obesity-diabetes-artery disease epidemic:
- Healthy joints support healthy muscles.
- Healthy muscles in frequent use support healthy metabolism.
- Healthy metabolism helps prevent abdominal obesity, prediabetes, and type 2 diabetes.
- Avoiding abdominal obesity, prediabetes, and type 2 diabetes helps support healthy arteries.
- Healthy arteries support a healthy heart and a healthy brain; that is a healthy and fun life!

Diabetes: type 1, type 2, or prediabetes?

What is diabetes?

Diabetes is diagnosed when blood sugar levels rise above the normal limit of about 100 mg/dl. When you say diabetes, think insulin, as the development of diabetes is closely related to problems with insulin, the hormone that allows blood sugar to enter the cells. Most common problems with insulin that lead to diabetes are:

- Inadequate insulin production by the pancreas beta cells
- Reduced insulin effect on the cells, mainly in the muscles and liver ("insulin resistance")
- Combination of the above, with both insufficient insulin production and reduced insulin effectiveness

What makes diabetes a dreaded "dis-ease" that it is is that the entire metabolism—not just carbs—is thrown up in chaos, creating a most "polluted" and unhealthy environment for all the cells and organs in our bodies as:

- **Sugar** piles up to unnaturally high levels in the bloodstream while cells are starving for energy (sugar can't get in due to problems with insulin)
- Cells need to turn to **fat** to meet their energy needs, causing equally unnatural high-fat trafficking

The combo of **high levels of sugar and fat in the bloodstream** sets the stage for **widespread organ damage**, leading, over the years, to the many and fearsome diabetes complications: artery diseases, like heart attacks, stroke, and leg amputations, but also kidney failure, blindness, and nerve damage.

Type 1 diabetes (the least common form and the one that is not related to obesity) is usually caused by an abrupt annihilation of our pancreas beta cells by "friendly fire." In a turn of bad luck, an otherwise mundane viral infection changes the "appearance" of the beta cells to our defence forces that see them as "invaders." **Friendly fire** then **destroys** those **beta cells**, reducing insulin production to almost zero. The situation is so dramatic that, unless the affected individual is treated with insulin, life ends quickly. Type 1 diabetes can affect individuals of any age (including children and young adults), even those who are thin and fit. Type 1 diabetes is not a part of the obesity-diabetes-artery disease epidemic. Once type 1 diabetic, you are likely to need insulin for the rest of your life.

Type 2 diabetes is altogether a different story. Not only is it the most common type of diabetes, it is also the one associated with obesity and the driving force behind the current obesity-diabetes-artery disease epidemic. Usually, type 2 diabetes develops slowly, over the course of several years to decades, in two stages:

- Stage 1: **abdominal obesity** floods our critical organs and muscle with fat and leads to i**nsulin resistance**, demanding increased insulin production from the beta cells.
- Stage 2: Beta cells, over the years, and especially in those with a first degree relative with type 2 diabetes, **start dying** off, exhausted by the increasing demands of insulin production (imposed by insulin resistance) and strangled by local pancreas fat, which normally has no place inside the pancreas.

Abdominal obesity and family history of type 2 diabetes are critical factors in developing this type of diabetes. As discussed before, once you have belly fat, there is **fat inside your critical organs**, including your liver ("fatty liver," under continuous shelling of fat through the unique belly fat-liver connection, the portal vein) and your muscles. This fat reduces the ability of your cells to take up sugar from the blood, in spite of normal or even high levels of insulin ("**insulin resistance**"). Inside your pancreas, this abnormally present fat strangles and suffocates the beta cells, reducing their capacity to produce insulin. So what starts insidiously, with just a little bit of belly fat, over several years to a few decades (the younger you are and the healthier your pancreas is, the longer it takes), becomes prediabetes or type 2 diabetes. In early years, type 2 diabetes appears to be a little more than a blood sugar problem, but later on the disease is defined by its complications:

- Artery disease ("macrovascular" complications, like heart attacks, stroke, leg and brain artery cholesterol plaques)
- "Microvascular" complications (kidney, eye and nerve damage)

In both types of diabetes, cell and organ damage are the end results of too much sugar ("**glucose toxicity**") and too much fat ("**lipotoxicity**") in the bloodstream and around our cells.

Prediabetes is a condition where blood sugar levels are higher than normal but lower than the sugar levels that define diabetes. It is a transitional state between healthy carb metabolism and type 2 diabetes (usually there is no prediabetes in type 1 diabetes). Prediabetes is, unfortunately, very common and affects one in three US adults. Risk factors for developing prediabetes include:

- Belly fat
- Family history of type 2 diabetes
- Sitting for too many hours every day and not moving around enough
- Getting older

Racial background and ethnicity also affect your risk of becoming prediabetic. The risk is lowest in non-hispanic whites and is higher in most other races in the US (African Americans, Hispanics, Asian Americans, Native Americans, and Pacific Islanders).

It is important to consider that both belly fat and prediabetes suggest "insulin resistance," which is the reduced ability of our bodies' cells (especially muscle, liver, and fat) to take up and use sugar, in spite of normal or even high amounts of insulin in the bloodstream. Insulin resistance challenges our pancreas beta cells, demanding increased insulin production to keep blood sugar levels normal. Over the years, especially in individuals with genetically less durable beta cells (for example, in those with family history of type 2 diabetes), beta cells get exhausted. In combination with beta cell exhaustion, abnormally placed local pancreas fat strangles the beta cells, leading to their demise. When most of the beta cells are gone, insulin production drops and blood sugar rises. This is diabetes.

Complications: the other face of diabetes

Whether type 1 or type 2, diabetes that has not been treated adequately will hurt your body, after granting you a grace period of about 5–8 years. There are two main types of diabetes complications, those that affect:

- Your larger arteries, leading to heart attacks, stroke, and clogged leg arteries and amputations ("macrovascular" complications)
- The smaller arteries that make up the filtering units of your kidneys, or the arteries that feed your eye's retina and your nerves ("microvascular" complications), potentially leading to kidney failure, blindness, or nerve malfunction, including burning pains in your feet and legs, interfering with night sleep

Diabetes also has a direct damaging effect on the heart muscle, making it stiff and unable to relax well and accommodate the incoming, oxygen-rich blood from the lungs. This is called "diastolic dysfunction," a very common process that, initially, results in shortness of breath. Over time, diabetes can also weaken the heart. We call this condition "diabetic cardiomyopathy," and it can result in heart failure and irregular heart rhythms like atrial fibrillation.

Controlling the blood sugar levels is a must for all diabetics. Out of control blood sugar will not only throw your metabolism up in chaos, but it will also lead to microvascular complications (kidney, eye, and nerve damage). However, in order to avoid heart attacks, stroke, and sudden death (the macrovascular complications—all forms of artery disease—that kill 85% of diabetics), **blood sugar control is not enough**. Strict blood pressure control (maintaining it no higher than 140/90 mmHg; some scientists advocate to keep BP less than 130/80, especially in diabetics younger than 60 years) and, above all, keeping the LDL—the bad cholesterol—low (below 70–100 mg/dl, depending on the circumstances) are necessary. A low-dose aspirin (81–100 mg a day) is recommended for many type 2 diabetics (in the absence of contraindications like stomach ulcers, stomach bleeding, and aspirin allergy) in order to prevent abnormal artery clotting (the final blow in a heart attack or a stroke). Finally, medications like lisinopril (or other "ACE-inhibitors") or losartan (or other "ARBs") have been shown to protect the kidneys of diabetics from failing and are also indicated for complication prevention in diabetes, even in the absence of high blood pressure.

The decision to start (and usually maintain for life) those medications that can prevent diabetes complications should be made jointly with your doctor, after considering all factors (including both the benefit and the potential for side effects) and with periodic blood testing to make sure your body tolerates these medications well. The importance of lifelong use of medications in diabetes for purposes other that blood sugar control is huge and too often is met with unyielding resistance by patients who focus on side effects without considering the benefit of prevention of deadly diabetes complications.

As type 2 diabetes is, in a large part, a lifestyle-related disease, a disciplined lifestyle is a must. Medications alone cannot compensate for smoking, lack of daily aerobic activity and frequent strengthening exercises, or a careless diet with bad carbs ("high glycemic index" carbs) or bad fats (saturated or trans fats). See Chapter 5 for details on healthy lifestyle.

High blood pressure

Blood pressure (BP) is the pressure exerted by the blood on the main artery, the aorta. As the main part of the heart (left ventricle) contracts, the aortic valve, the door that separates the heart from the aorta, opens and about two to three ounces of blood rush into the aorta. The aorta is the main artery superhighway that starts at the heart and, by dividing into smaller and smaller branches, reaches all the cells in our body. The blood in the aorta is under tension, a driving force that propels the blood to the furthest corner of our body. The tension in the aorta (that is, the blood pressure) is higher at the time that the heart contracts ("systole") and blood rushes into the aorta; this BP is called systolic BP (top number). It is lower when the heart relaxes (diastolic BP or low/bottom number).

The absolutely perfect systolic BP (top number) is 90–115 mmHg; the absolutely perfect diastolic BP (low or bottom number) is 70–79 mmHg. It used to be that medications for high BP were not prescribed unless it was higher than 140/90 mmHg. In 2017, two important scientific organizations (American College of Cardiology and American Heart Association) changed the thresholds to 130/80 mmHg. Under this definition of high BP ("hypertension"), almost one in two adult Americans has high blood pressure.

High blood pressure is dangerous because it can cause heart and artery damage; heart attacks, stroke, heart failure, and atrial fibrillation are among the major complications of high BP. It can also cause kidney and eye damage. Kidney disease, although it doesn't kill as quickly as a heart attack or a stroke, is the #9 killer disease in the US and an important result of the obesity-diabetes-artery disease epidemic, as high blood pressure (a frequent consequence of obesity) and diabetes are the primary causes of kidney disease. It is important to note that BP can be dangerously high (e.g., 200/100 mmHg) without causing absolutely any symptoms. This is why hypertension is frequently called the "silent killer." For the same reason, I recommend to all my patients to buy a BP machine and monitor their BP at least once a month, even if they never had any blood pressure issues. With the advent of childhood obesity, hypertension is now, unfortunately, diagnosed even in children and adolescents. The older we get, the higher the BP gets. It is estimated that almost 80–90 percent of individuals at the age of 80 years will have high BP.

High blood pressure is one of the most common reasons a patient sees his primary care provider or a specialist like a cardiologist or a nephrologist. The foundation of treating high blood pressure is sticking to a healthy lifestyle with special emphasis on losing weight and reducing the amount of salt and animal fat in your diet. If an attempt at healthy lifestyle does not get your BP below 130/80 mmHg, your doctor may prescribe a medication. Persuading a young person to start taking a pill for high blood pressure is frequently a difficult task. Young people think of themselves as young and healthy, and this image is literally shattered by the pill the doctor prescribes for high BP. Also, many patients (not only the young ones) focus more on the side effects of the medications and forget the "side effects" of high BP (heart attacks, stroke, heart failure, atrial fibrillation and kidney failure). It is also important to know that if you take NSAIDs (medications like ibuprofen or naproxen, Aleve or Advil—see Chapter 5) every day for a prolonged period of time (months or years), you may develop high BP and a host of other complications (heart attacks, heart failure, high potassium, fluid retention, stomach problems, and bleeding). Talk to your doctor if you take any of these medications.

Metabolic and cardiometabolic syndrome

The **metabolic syndrome i**s frequently the common denominator in individuals affected by the obesity-diabetes-artery disease epidemic. While the scientific criteria for its diagnosis are complex and vary among different organizations, in simpler terms metabolic syndrome implies the presence of belly fat along with some of the key features of **insulin resistance** like:

- Abnormally high blood sugar (prediabetes or type 2 diabetes)
- High triglycerides or low HDL (the good cholesterol) or
- High blood pressure

As these metabolic abnormalities set the stage for the development of widespread cholesterol plaques in our arteries (artery disease resulting in heart attacks or heart failure) or directly damage the heart (by making it stiff—"diastolic dysfunction"—or weak), the term "**cardiometabolic syndrome**" ("cardia" is the greek word for heart) was also created. The concept of cardiometabolic syndrome emphasizes the link between an abnormal metabolism, on the one hand, and artery and heart disease, on the other, and explains the addition of the term "artery disease" in the "obesity-diabetes-artery disease" epidemic.

Disease is often the combination of a bad lifestyle, bad genes, and time passing by. Some of these factors we can change, but some others we cannot, like our genetics and our age. For this reason, aging is a huge force that we all must reckon with.

Does every obese person have an abnormal metabolism?

The answer is "No." Where scientists disagree is how often this does happen and whether normal metabolism is maintained in the long run.

A "metabolically healthy obese" (MHO) individual is someone who is classified as obese by BMI or waist circumference criteria, while he has none of the metabolic abnormalities associated with obesity. Such a person is expected to have all of the features below:

- Normal blood pressure (by most recent definition: below 130/80 mmHg)
- Normal triglycerides (below 150 mg/dl)
- Normal HDL (at least 40 mg/dl for men and 50 mg/dl for women)

- Normal fasting blood sugar (99 mg/dl or lower), meaning no diabetes or prediabetes
- Normal A1c (5.6% or lower)

A metabolically healthy obese person should try to maintain all the features of normal metabolism in the long run, as the effects of obesity on metabolism can take several years to develop.

How frequent is it to find such a person? Here there is wide disagreement between scientists, as every scientific group uses different criteria for defining who is a MHO. Some scientists suggest that almost half of the obese individuals have no metabolic problems; they admit though that, over the ensuing five to six years of follow up, almost one half of these MHO start showing up signs of abnormal metabolism. Some other scientific studies suggest that the condition of MHO is rare. One such study followed MHO for nine years. At the end of the study, only 1.3% of those maintained a normal metabolism.

Change and aging

As we age, we change. While aging to many young people means grey hair and skin wrinkles, it is the effects on other organs systems like muscle, fat, bone, and arteries that are associated with aging-related disease. With aging we gain fat and lose muscle and bone. Our metabolism slows down. Joint cartilage is damaged and is not regenerated, contributing to arthritis that reduces our mobility, further slowing down our metabolism. Abdominal obesity and aging bring fat inside and around our heart, arteries, liver, pancreas, and muscle. This abnormally placed fat is a poison to the organs that host it. For example, the presence of fat inside the pancreas kills the insulin-producing beta cells and contributes to the development of type 2 diabetes, which becomes more common the older we get. Fat in the heart contributes to diastolic dysfunction (stiffening of the heart muscle) and atrial fibrillation (a stroke-prone irregular heart rhythm, common after the age of 65). Fat around our arteries contributes to atherosclerosis (cholesterol plaque development inside the arteries, the precursor of heart attacks and stroke). Aging also causes a proinflammatory condition with a lingering and mild but widespread inflammation that contributes to artery and heart disease, cancer, and arthritis. A final and inescapable fact about aging is that it is programmed in our genes and, up to now, the elixir of youth has not been found, in spite of intense and ongoing scientific efforts.

Whether a man or a woman, it is impossible to be 60 years old and look, feel, or perform like you did when you were 20. However, there are people who age well, staying functional and independent and enjoying life well into their eighties, and there are others who age badly, developing crippling knee arthritis because of obesity and weak muscles, emphysema because of smoking, or heart failure because of high blood pressure or diabetes. It is up to us to concede the absolute minimum losses to aging. In the area of muscle loss, for example, there is strong scientific evidence that resistance exercises, when practiced frequently, can help us not only avoid muscle loss but also gain muscle in spite of aging. Some may think that more muscle simply means a better appearance, but the real benefits of well-developed and maintained muscle are a faster and more robust metabolism and physical independence, without the need for knee replacement surgery, falls, a cane, a walker, or a nursing home placement. Healthy diet and exercise also reduce risk for Alzheimer's and depression, boosting further our independence and functionality later in life. Decent genes, a healthy lifestyle, and a little bit of luck can win you independence and good performance well into your late eighties. On the other hand, a heavy smoker with belly fat who spends most of his or her day sitting and eating bad carbs and bad fats can miss quite a bit, as death can strike swiftly in the form of a heart attack in his forties (men) or her fifties (women), even if such a person is endowed with decent genes. So, live well and age better!

Health care or "sick care"?

When we talk of "healthcare," we intuitively think of hospitals, doctors, and nurses treating people who are sick. And we also think, of course, of "healthcare insurance," painfully reminded to all of us by skyrocketing premiums and deductibles. But is this right? Shouldn't we be calling the care that is delivered by doctors and nurses to people who suffer from disease "sick care"? And the insurance that covers such expenses "sick-care insurance"? And if so, what is the true meaning of "healthcare" and "healthcare insurance"?

To be fair to all parts, there are those wellness visits to primary care doctors and other providers, and these are true "healthcare." During these visits your healthcare provider discusses prevention and wellness issues with you, reviews necessary immunizations, and goes over important biometrics like your blood pressure, blood sugar and A1c (a measure of your long-term blood sugar levels), your cholesterol numbers (LDL—the bad cholesterol, HDL—the good cholesterol and triglycerides), your TSH (reflects thyroid function), creatinine (kidney function), and hemoglobin. And many insurances support wellness programs that motivate their insured individuals to take steps to keep them well.

On the other hand, and in the context of the obesity-diabetes-artery disease epidemic, being treated for a heart attack, stroke, heart failure, or any other diabetes complication is "disease care" or "sick care," not health care. The most you can hope for from the best hospital and doctors is minimizing your health losses from your heart attack or stroke. And rehab will try to get you in shape after such an event, something that prevention and wellness specialists has been begging you to do before you got ill. Isn't it petty to wait until you lose half your heart or a big chunk of your brain before you decide to change your lifestyle? Your best health insurance is investing in wellness and prevention as early in life as possible. See what tricks you can pick up by reading the rest of this book. However, for the sake of your health, be sure to skip Chapter 3.

Chapter 2 Questions

Invest in your people's health, not just their education.

1. Which of the following is not part of the metabolic syndrome?
   a. Smoking
   b. High blood pressure
   c. High triglycerides
   d. Prediabetes

2. Is it possible to find fat in between heart muscle cells?

3. Why are pancreas beta cells so important?

4. How frequent is fatty liver?

5. In our forties, many of us subject to a Western lifestyle have cholesterol plaques in the walls of our arteries. How can these plaques be "flushed out"?

6. Diabetes causes our blood sugar to be high, and this is dangerous for our health. What else, beyond high blood sugar, makes diabetes a life-threatening disease?

7. The cell is the unit of life. Even if one out of the 37 trillion cells in our body undergoes a change, our body is different. How quickly can a cell change?

8. A stable cholesterol plaque in the wall of our arteries may never cause any health problem or symptom. Once that same plaque becomes unstable, though, a clot can be formed over the plaque and completely clog the artery, potentially causing a heart attack, a stroke, or sudden death. How quickly can a clot form over an unstable cholesterol plaque?

9. What type of diabetes is associated with obesity?

10. What is more common?
    a. Type 1 diabetes
    b. Type 2 diabetes
    c. Prediabetes

Chapter 3

THE PATH TO AN UNHEALTHY LIFESTYLE

"Most people have no idea how good their body is designed to feel."
—Kevin Trudeau

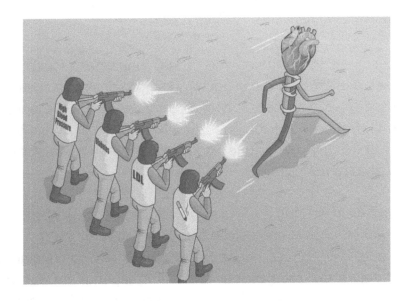

A Guide to Artery Destruction

Suppose you want to commit suicide but you hate cliches. Using a gun, jumping off a cliff, or taking a drug overdose is simply not you. You want to try something different and out of the ordinary. You hear left and right about heart disease being the #1 killer, and you want to experience the hype. You might have read the previous chapters and been intrigued about the "obesity-diabetes-artery disease epidemic." So, you decide to die by destroying your arteries. You are determined to do whatever it takes to succeed, but since you haven't done it before, you need some guidance. Dying by destroying your arteries is not as simple as buying a gun and a bullet and pulling the trigger. You need to make long-range plans, execute them carefully, and be patient. Before you start, you need to know roughly how long it will take, what your checklist should be, and what you should expect along the way. This chapter will answer your questions and help you design the perfect artery self-destruction adventure that will keep you engaged to the very end.

As you cannot see your arteries, you cannot simply get a weapon, aim at your arteries, and shoot at them. So, how can you destroy something that you can't see? A valid strategy is by delivering your lethal weapons inside your arteries. But how can you do this? What are the weapons that have the power to destroy your arteries, and what are the means of deploying those weapons to the frontlines?

In Chapter 2 we described arteries as an intricate network of smart tubes that start from the heart and deliver blood-carrying oxygen and nutrients to all our cells in all our organs. **As all our organs rely on constant blood delivery through our arteries, our entire life depends on our arteries.** When blood stops flowing, our cells and organs start dying, some within minutes, some others within hours. Anything that would impair the constant delivery of blood through our arteries can result in death. That's why you can kill yourself by destroying your arteries! And it is the obesity-diabetes-heart disease epidemic that will provide you the best tools to get the job done.

Arteries are hard at work 24/7 and suffer quite a bit of wear and tear along the way. For this reason, the most intuitive and common-sense approach to damaging your arteries (short of cutting them open with a knife) is by speeding up their "natural" wear and tear. Think of artery wear and tear as road damage; while rare car traffic in places without extreme temperatures will take years to cause significant road damage, a more frequent, near constant traffic of heavy vehicles along with extreme temperatures (regular freezing and salting of the road to prevent icing), can damage even a well-built road in only a few months. For the arteries, wear and tear comes in the form of cholesterol plaques in the artery walls ("atherosclerosis"). Cholesterol plaques are so common that most of us (especially men) have some cholesterol plaques in our arteries by our late twenties/early thirties. Cholesterol plaque formation is the artery's way of healing the many daily micro-damages it is subjected to in the form of:

- "Shear stress" of blood flowing under pressure inside them and "scratching" the artery wall or "hitting" the divider wall (tee) at the site of an artery bifurcation into smaller branches
- The stress of conforming to the movement of the organ the particular arteries serve, being most conspicuous for the heart arteries (heart arteries turn and squeeze about 100,000 times a day following a movement akin to wringing a wet towel)

Cholesterol plaques usually do not directly hurt us, as, when quiet and stable, they leave plenty of room for the blood to flow. What makes cholesterol plaques potential killers is their ability, when mature, to change quickly and incite clots. Mature cholesterol plaques can instantly—and unpredictably—become unstable, provoking blood clotting that can completely clog the artery, within only one to four minutes. A clogged heart artery may mean a heart attack or sudden death; a clogged brain artery may result in a stroke or sudden death. The "normal" artery wear and tear will take many decades to kill you; you will be probably in your late seventies before you see your "dream" of death by artery destruction come true. But wait, there are plenty of tried and proven ways you can accelerate the wear and tear process and drop dead from a heart attack as early as in your mid thirties, although individual results may vary. You want early and deadly artery destruction, and we will help you achieve it. So, how can you help create more of those cholesterol plaques in the walls of your arteries, and how can you turn them deadly?

Cholesterol is necessary for life as cholesterol makes up:
- Part of the cell wall (cell "membrane")
- Hormones
- Vitamin D
- Bile

However, this does not mean that we need to eat foods rich in cholesterol, as our liver is capable of making as much cholesterol as we need from scratch. Cholesterol made by the liver travels through the bloodstream to reach cells anywhere in the body. Cholesterol, though, is fat, while blood is water-based; thus, cholesterol cannot be dissolved in the blood. Instead, special shuttles called lipoproteins (both LDL and HDL are such shuttles) are used to transport cholesterol in the bloodstream (they are made of protein on the outside that can mix with blood and cholesterol on the inside). For the modern person, the amount of cholesterol in the bloodstream usually exceeds what is considered healthy.

Also, for the modern person with abdominal obesity, belly fat transforms the liver into "fatty liver," a factory of artery destruction. Fatty liver churns up LDL models that are smaller and more dangerous. Under these circumstances, LDL cholesterol does its diabolic magic: while circulating in the bloodstream, it passes vertically through the artery lining and gets trapped inside the artery wall. This is the first step in the formation of cholesterol plaque ("fatty streaks"). Later on, trapped LDL attracts inflammation, with some of the inflammatory cells eating up LDL and becoming "foam cells" that cause even more inflammation. And while inflammation as a process can provide protection against invaders and other threats, the inflammation inside cholesterol plaques is a "non-resolving," never-ending, and destructive process that, decades after it first started, can incite clot formation. **The clot on top of an unstable cholesterol plaque is the final event in this type of artery disease and can clog the artery within a few minutes, resulting in strokes or heart attacks.** Finally, HDL, the good cholesterol, plays an important role in cholesterol plaque disease (atherosclerosis). HDL removes cholesterol from the artery wall and returns it to the liver. The higher the HDL, the less aggressive artery cholesterol plaques become and the lower the risk of heart attacks and stroke. Therefore, the recipe for suicide by way of artery destruction is:

- Get as much LDL cholesterol as possible into your bloodstream.
- Gain belly fat so that your liver becomes "fatty liver" and starts making LDL models that are more destructive than usual.
- Do whatever it takes (e.g., smoking or developing high blood pressure) to promote not only the formation of more cholesterol plaques inside your arteries but also the maturation and instability of those plaques so that clot is formed on top of the plaque and clogs the artery. You already know what follows: heart attack, stroke, or sudden death.
- Do whatever it takes to lower your HDL (smoke cigarettes, do not exercise, gain weight, eat plenty of trans fats and bad sugars).

While LDL level is influenced by heredity, age, gender, obesity, and other risk factors for artery disease (like high blood pressure), there are a lot of things we can do to make artery disease worse.

Question: How do we get our blood LDL cholesterol high?

Answer:
- Eating more saturated fats (red meat, cold cuts, whole fat dairy, baked goods, processed foods, french fries, buffalo wings, pizza, and other fast foods).
- Eating more trans fats (deep-fried and processed foods).
- Eating more calories and exercising less so that we become overweight or obese; belly fat will take care of the rest.
- Reducing body movement and exercise as much as possible; sitting 12 hours a day and absolutely no exercise will do.
- Refusing any statins or other cholesterol-lowering medications your doctor may want to prescribe for you. Refraining from visiting your doctor altogether is an even better strategy for developing early and life-threatening artery disease.
- Being chronically sleep deprived.

Question: How do we gain belly fat?

Answer:
- Reducing body movement and exercise as much as possible; sitting 12 hours a day and absolutely no exercise will do.
- Eating more calories and exercising less, so that we can become overweight; high-calorie foods, like bad fats and bad carbs, will help you consume as many calories as possible. Bad carbs are particularly helpful in order to gain weight, as they cause insulin to spike; this makes you slightly hypoglycemic less than two hours after you eat them, so you feel hungry and eat again. White bread, white pasta, cookies, desserts, cakes, candies, donuts, and sugary beverages are great at making you hungry quickly and forcing you to eat again.
- Refraining from fruits and vegetables, as they have few calories and, instead, they contain fiber that helps you avoid insulin spikes. That means that fruits and vegetables may keep you satisfied for three to five hours after you've eaten them and reduce the overall amount of food and calories you consume. They make it harder to develop belly fat. They also contain antioxidants that protect your arteries against cholesterol plaque disease.
- Stinting on sleep. Sleeping less than seven hours per night increases your appetite, leading you to become overweight or obese. It also increases the levels of cortisol, one of the "stress hormones" that can make you prediabetic. It also increases your blood pressure and bad cholesterol (LDL) and triglycerides and reduces your good cholesterol (HDL).

Question: How do we, otherwise, increase our risk for artery disease?

Answer:
- Smoking
- Developing High Blood Pressure
- Developing type 2 Diabetes
- Using NSAIDs (medications like ibuprofen, naproxen, Advil, or Aleve, see also Chapter 5) every day for many months or years

Smoking contains 7,000 chemicals. Many of these chemicals damage the lining of your arteries ("endothelium"), increasing LDL trapping and inflammation inside the artery wall and contributing to the formation, maturation, and instability of cholesterol plaques. Smoking also reduces your good cholesterol (HDL).

High blood pressure also damages the artery lining and promotes the formation, maturation, and instability of cholesterol plaques. It can also destroy your arteries by causing aneurysms. When aneurysms rupture suddenly, death is likely unless emergency medical care is sought.

Type 2 diabetes damages the arteries in many ways, by:
- Damaging the lining of the arteries ("endothelium")
- Making clots more likely to form
- Worsening the damaging effect of LDL, the bad cholesterol

There are also the direct effects of increased belly fat, present in about 90 percent of patients with type 2 diabetes. Belly fat means insulin resistance and fatty liver (the liver making more destructive LDL models). In diabetes, there are also abnormally high levels of trafficking of both sugar (glucose) and fat molecules. This "cocktail" is toxic to all cells and accounts for many of the diabetes complications (artery disease, like heart attacks and stroke, and also kidney, eye, and nerve damage).

As we have discussed in the previous paragraph, the secret behind artery damage is accelerating the normal artery wear and tear. In the road damage metaphor, rare car traffic in places with mild temperatures is not very damaging. However, a more frequent, near constant traffic of heavy vehicles along with extreme temperatures can damage even a well-built road in only a few months. What is heavy traffic to road damage is high blood pressure and high cholesterol to artery damage. And what is extreme temperatures and salting to the road is smoking and diabetes to your arteries. This is why accelerated artery damage flourishes under conditions of:
- High blood pressure
- High cholesterol
- Smoking
- Diabetes

You want early and advanced artery damage? Here is your checklist of things you should be doing on a daily basis:

- Eat as much as you can. Choose saturated and trans fats (red meat, fried and fast foods, processed foods, cold cuts, whole fat milk, and cheese) and bad carbs (cookies, desserts, candies, donuts, ice cream, milk chocolate, cakes, white bread, and white pasta), lots of them. By doing so you help both your blood cholesterol and blood pressure to go up. And you are on the right path to becoming diabetic.
- Stay away from fruits, vegetables, whole grains, and oatmeal. All these types of food can lower your cholesterol (these foods contain little or no cholesterol, and fiber in them will reduce cholesterol absorption) and blood pressure (through increased potassium intake and lower body weight). They can also delay the development of diabetes (through delayed absorption of bad "high glycemic index" carbs—see previous bullet point—and by not being calorie-dense).
- Exercise for as little as it is necessary to get by. Sit for a minimum of 8 hours every day (12 hours is even better). Grab every sitting opportunity you can: at home, at work, while commuting, in front of your TV or computer screen. Play lots of computer games in a relaxed, seated position. Do not try any treadmill desks or standing desks, and don't exercise while watching TV. Think of exercise as your enemy in achieving artery destruction. Sitting will help you increase your body weight and your blood pressure, and cholesterol and will increase the chances of developing type 2 diabetes. Sitting will help you retain stress (as opposed to exercise), which will lead you to eat higher quantities of bad carbs and bad fats.
- Smoke every day. Don't worry if you do not like cigarettes. Smoke cigars, vapor, e-cigarettes, hookah, marijuana, anything will do (smoking any of these substances is likely to damage the artery lining endothelium, raise your blood pressure, reduce your good cholesterol—HDL—and increase the chance of becoming diabetic).
- Do anything possible to increase the amount of belly fat (items #1 and #2 are key).
- Do anything possible to become type 2 diabetic (all items above).

- Do anything possible to get your blood pressure high (increase your belly fat, increase salt intake, reduce exercise, increase saturated fats, reduce potassium intake, and increase your stress level).
- Sleep less than seven hours per night, work third shift, and work more than 55 hours per week. All these will help destroy your arteries through high blood pressure, abnormal sugar metabolism, or stroke. Your hunger increases, and you are more likely to consume "comfort food" like the bad carbs of the first bullet point.
- Consume ibuprofen, naproxen, Advil, Aleve, or any other NSAIDs on a daily basis, even if you don't have pains or arthritis. Instead of using diphenhydramine alone to help you sleep, use it in combination with the NSAIDs (like ibuprofen PM, naproxen PM, Advil PM, or Aleve PM).
- Abuse alcohol.

Heart attacks: how they happen

The way to damage our arteries starts by damaging their inner lining, those special "endothelial" cells. Endothelial cells are endowed with a host of unique properties, but what is most relevant to our discussion is that, unless they form a healthy and robust carpet that covers and seals the entire inner surface of all of our arteries, the blood that flows over them will clot and clog the artery. The usual scenario of such a thing happening is when a mature cholesterol plaque "cracks." A mature cholesterol plaque contains a diverse population of cells and chemical materials (including cholesterol). The plaque's top layer is formed, among others, by endothelial cells that coat and seal the plaque's entire surface, without leaving any gaps. As a result, the flowing blood stays separate from the plaque. If and when such a plaque becomes instantly and unpredictably unstable, cracks develop in its cap, and gaps appear among the endothelial cells that cover the plaque.

This is all it takes to get the artery clogged in just a few minutes: as the blood that flows over the plaque is exposed to the inner materials of the cholesterol plaque, blood interprets the situation as if the artery is damaged and bleeding. The blood then, as is programmed to do under such circumstances, forms a clot. But this clot doesn't seal a hole in a bleeding artery; instead, it clogs a previously open artery and stops the blood flow.

The result is quick death of the cells that depend on that artery. When this happens in a heart artery, the result is a heart attack or sudden death. When it happens in a brain artery, the result is a stroke or sudden death.

Killing your arteries: your final moments

So, you have been a dedicated artery killer and have been trying consistently for years to get this job well done. You did most of the things we mentioned: you have been a daily, heavy smoker (for the purpose of artery disease, more than two cigarettes a day makes you a heavy smoker) with a profound aversion to any form of exercise, a devoted supporter of sitting as the default human position, an avid consumer of cookies, candies, donuts, desserts, and cakes, a frequent customer of fast food, an alcohol abuser, a third shift worker, a daily consumer of naproxen or ibuprofen, a workaholic, and sleep-stinter. You have seen, over the years, your waistline grow, your blood pressure, LDL cholesterol, and triglycerides rise, your A1c in the diabetic range; you know you are on the right path to artery destruction. You know the final act will be quick. And you have been patiently waiting for this ultimate thrill. Here are a few common scenarios that demonstrate how your final moments are likely to be, while a clot starts forming over an unstable cholesterol plaque in one of your heart or brain arteries:

- A rough day at work, your boss demanding more from you, with suffocating deadlines and the implicit threat that you might be losing your job if you do not meet them. You tough it out with a few cigarettes and alcohol. You go to bed, but bad thoughts are in your mind. You die in your sleep around 4:30 a.m.
- Your day has been fine, so far. Suddenly, you feel some heaviness in your chest that grows quickly in intensity. You do nothing. 30 minutes later, you start perspiring and feel you are dying. Although your wish was to die by artery destruction, you feel scared now, so you call 911. In the emergency department, they give you an aspirin, some pills, and a morphine injection. ER pages the interventional cardiologist on call. Your heart rhythm, as seen in your monitor, deteriorates. You hear your nurse: "VT. Call a code; get the defibrillator ready." You then lose consciousness.

- Your blood pressure is 210/120; you take no medications. Unexpectedly, you feel a tearing chest pain and, moments later, you pass out.
- You are out partying; It has been a blast! You had so much fun and so much to eat and drink. You smoked a couple of cigars and are now dancing. All of a sudden, you develop a cold sweat, start vomiting, and get dizzy. Last thing in your memory: your friends were laying you down on the sofa.
- You are in your car driving. Stuck in traffic. You are late and stressed. You light a cigarette. Minutes later, you can't breathe and your left arm hurts. Then everything goes blank.

Killing your arteries: a year earlier

- You were diagnosed with type 2 diabetes several years ago. You do take your blood sugar pills. Your doctor has recommended a statin and an aspirin, which you, of course, have refused to take. After some research that you did over the internet, you find out that statins have so many potential side effects; they can kill your liver, your muscles, and your kidneys. However, statins are great at protecting your arteries, which is exactly what you have been trying to avoid.
- Your blood pressure has been consistently around 160/95. You want to destroy your arteries, so this blood pressure suits you just fine. You have repeatedly refused taking any blood pressure medications. On top of saving your life by preventing artery damage, these pills are loaded with undesirable side effects (dizziness, sexual dysfunction, a dry cough, kidney problems, ankle swelling, dry mouth, fatigue, or even depression). So, it's a no brainer: blood pressure pills are a no-no for you.
- After smoking for about thirty years, you have developed emphysema and were forced to cut down. You now only smoke three or four cigarettes a day. You want to tear down your arteries, but you don't want to die from emphysema. Emphysema makes your breathing so difficult and heavy that the simple act of breathing feels like drowning. Emphysema is a torture, in spite of the oxygen tank you carry everywhere you go. You think that by cutting down

the number of the cigarettes you smoke you will slow down the process of lung destruction. You can't take any worsening of your breathing. You have also heard that two cigarettes a day are still capable of causing heart attacks. For you, a heart attack a better way to go than emphysema. Besides, this is what you wanted in the first place.

- You are severely overweight and prediabetic. Your knees hurt. You start taking ibuprofen 600 mg three times a day. Your knee pain is better. Kidney function is borderline. You have heard that NSAIDs can cause heart attacks, if taken frequently. You want to destroy your arteries, so daily ibuprofen is just fine. At night, you use ibuprofen PM (ibuprofen+diphenhydramine). It helps you sleep, although diphenhydramine without the ibuprofen would have helped you sleep exactly the same way.

Killing your arteries: a decade earlier

- You are overweight but not yet obese. You used to go to the gym every other day but have learned that frequent exercise can help prevent heart disease and diabetes. So you cancel your gym membership.
- Your spouse complains that you never eat any fruits or vegetables. Your waist circumference is 48 inches. You have never told her you want to commit suicide by wrecking your arteries.
- Your mom had type 2 diabetes. You do not exercise and eat a donut every day. You drink a couple of sugary colas with lunch and a bottle of wine with dinner. Your A1c is 6.3%, in the prediabetic range, so you know you are on the right path.
- Your LDL is 210 (mg/dl). A high-dose statin has caused muscle cramps. Your dad and your sister both had heart attacks, in their forties and fifties, respectively. There are some newer cholesterol medications, but they are too expensive.
- You are a workaholic. You are driven by success at all costs. You believe that sleeping longer than five hours a night is a waste of time. You have no time to exercise. You smoke cigars regularly. There is a lot on your mind; stress is a daily factor. But that's good; you want to kill your arteries, don't you?

- You snore at night and feel unrefreshed during the day. Your doctor suspects obstructive sleep apnea. She counsels you that sleep apnea is a serious health problem and, among other complications, it can make your blood pressure go very high. And high blood pressure can destroy your heart and your arteries. That's good news for you. You don't tell your doctor, but you are not going to go for the sleep study or, if your sleep breathing is abnormal, start wearing a special mask during your sleep.
- Your doctor just told you you are now officially a diabetic (type 2)! Inconvenient, yes, but surely a stepping stone in destroying your arteries. You are dining out tonight to celebrate this good news. White pasta, no salad, and, of course, a dessert at the end.

Chapter 3 Questions

1. Match the following terms:
   a. Endothelium
   b. Atherosclerosis
   c. Diastolic Dysfunction
   d. Complex movement like wringing a wet towel

with:

   A. Development of cholesterol plaques in the artery wall
   B. Inner lining of the arteries
   C. The arteries of the heart
   D. Stiff heart

2. What number of cigarettes per day is safe for our arteries?

3. Can we survive with zero cholesterol in our body?

4. Which of the following scenarios is more likely to kill a person by destroying his or her arteries?
   a. High blood pressure in her sixties
   b. Type 2 diabetes and smoking in his forties
   c. High triglycerides in his thirties
   d. A 20-year old eats healthy and is a non-smoker but never exercises

5. You have a big belly (abdominal obesity), you eat cookies and cheeseburgers every day, you never exercise, and you only sleep four to five hours per night. What else can you do to quicken the development of killer cholesterol plaques in your arteries?

6. What symptoms are you most likely to develop if your heart arteries have numerous cholesterol plaques that cause less than 50 percent artery narrowing?

7. How can you tell whether a chest discomfort that you are experiencing is due to acid reflux or a heart attack?

8. For the last two years you have been suffering from daily headaches, which you treat yourself with over-the-counter medications. You take two to three pills a day, depending on how bad your headaches are. Which one over-the-counter medication, when taken daily for that long a period of time (two years), is more likely to destroy your arteries?
   - Acetaminophen (brand name Tylenol)
   - Ibuprofen (brand names Advil and Motrin)

9. Small amounts of alcohol are good for your health. Large amounts of alcohol (three or more drinks per day for men up to the age of 65 or two or more drinks per day for women or men age 65 or older) will damage your arteries. How (through what mechanisms)?

10. You are destined to develop a large heart attack at age 42. One year earlier, what symptoms are most likely to be present and warn you of what is coming?

Chapter 4

THE PATH TO PREVENTION, HEALTH, PEACE & WELLNESS

*"Being healthy and fit isn't a fad or a trend.
It is a lifestyle."*
— Unknown

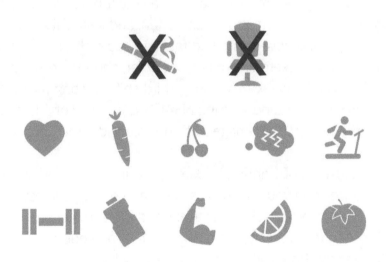

How to protect your arteries

Chapter 3 was about how to destroy one's arteries by accelerating their normal wear and tear; how to help cholesterol plaques form and develop in the artery wall silently for decades before they are mature enough to cause heart attacks or stroke; and how these plaques start inconspicuously in our early teens as "**fatty streaks,**" maturing slowly through our twenties and thirties as "**atherosclerotic plaques**" and, thereafter, getting ready to kill at a moment's notice. We learned about the importance of **endothelium**, the super smooth carpet that lines the inner surface of our arteries and how, under conditions conducive to artery destruction, this smooth barrier is penetrated by evil LDL molecules that end up making the artery wall their home. Then, LDL, permanently trapped in the artery wall, ignites a never ending inflammation that determines the pace of cholesterol plaque maturation and culminates in plaque instability and clot formation, which clogs the artery, causing heart attacks, stroke, or sudden death. We explained how smoking, high blood cholesterol, high blood pressure, and diabetes all contribute to artery destruction by accelerating the formation, maturation, and instability of cholesterol plaques. We explained how eating bad fats and bad carbs, sitting more than eight hours a day, not exercising, having belly fat, stinting on sleep, working more than 55 hours a week or working third shift, inviting as much stress as possible into our lives, and abusing NSAIDs is our way of adding insult to injury and furthering artery damage. Let's now consider the opposite.

Suppose that, instead of wanting to damage your arteries and shorten your life, you desire to keep your arteries as clean and free of cholesterol plaque as possible, avoid heart attacks and stroke, and live a longer and happier life without the need for heart bypass or brain artery procedures. What should you do? How early should you start your healthy lifestyle? And how is your everyday life likely to be? Is your life going to be a long but dull one, full of restrictions and devoid of fun? And by inverting the point made in the quest for artery destruction, how can you protect something you cannot even see?

Healthy metabolism means healthy arteries

Artery protection starts in places you wouldn't imagine have much to do with the health of your arteries. Artery health depends on healthy metabolism. Metabolism includes all these complex chemical transformations that take the energy from the food we eat and the drinks we drink and convert it to whatever function is necessary for our cells and body organs to survive and operate well: muscle movement, brain energy, food digestion, liver chemistry, heart pumping, bone formation, injury healing, and fighting invaders. Whatever keeps our metabolism healthy is the key to our artery health. And while our heredity, gender, and age are all major factors that affect our metabolism and are beyond our control, there is a lot we can do to keep our metabolism as robust and healthy as possible. Key among the positive actions we can take to improve our metabolism are:

- Using our muscles
- Burning calories
- Eating smart
- Sleeping adequately

Muscle and joints

Strong and active muscles speed up our metabolism and protect our arteries. And since muscle contraction requires healthy joints, the small and inconspicuous joint cartilage is also a vital—if indirect—part of our artery health; torn cartilage makes muscle movement painful and forces us to keep these muscles inactive, which slows down our metabolism and makes for unhealthy arteries. Also, joint arthritis may make us take medications like NSAIDs (see Chapter 6) that are directly damaging our arteries. So, artery protection needs strong muscles and healthy joints. Our body contains over 600 muscles, and muscle makes up more than a third to almost half of our body weight. All this muscle is there for a reason: to be used for several hours every day. Scientists believe that the physical activities for which the human body was built were those of the caveman. Paleo fitness, scientists estimate, consisted of two to four hours of moderate intensity cardio activity, complemented by lifting of heavy objects, pushing, tearing, and tree-climbing; in summary, Paleo fitness included several hours of combination exercise (aerobic, resistance, and stretching), seven days a week. How does this compare to what the modern man performs in the course of a day?

Adequate muscle activity supports and fosters a healthy metabolism. Not only does muscle burn calories when active, but it will continue burning extra calories for hours after muscle activity has stopped, even during sleep. So, keeping our muscles well developed, busy, and engaged throughout our daily activities is a key strategy to achieve a healthy metabolism. And for our muscles to move and work smoothly, our joints need to be healthy, as joint pain will prevent muscle use. I want you to keep in mind that:

- While strengthening exercises (like lifting weights) build muscle and support a healthy metabolism, lifting or pushing weights so heavy that it makes us strain while holding our breath ("isometric exercise with Valsalva maneuver") may dramatically increase our blood pressure to unhealthy levels. This extreme weight lifting can raise our blood pressure up to 300 mmHg; such a high blood pressure may be sustained for up to 20 minutes after we are done lifting. The human body was not made to withstand such excessive pressure inside its arteries. This is the reason many professional weightlifters and bodybuilders develop aneurysms of their chest ("thoracic") aorta, the major artery that starts in the heart and branches out to the rest of our body. A sudden burst of such an aneurysm may prove fatal.

- Very intense workouts are touted as helping you burn many calories and sculpt your body in a short period of time. I understand how difficult it may be to put aside adequate time for exercise in your busy schedule, but before picking up any form of exercise, ask yourself the question: **do my joints (back, knees, hip, shoulders) give me the green light** to go on with this type of exercise? Consider that some high-intensity exercises may put a lot of strain on your joints and result in injuries, eventually causing knee, back, hip, or shoulder arthritis. This is a big problem, as our joint cartilage does not regenerate beyond our late teens/early twenties. Once joint arthritis settles, it will stay there for the rest of our lives, and it usually gets worse as we age. Arthritis is a major factor of pain and disability after our fifties. Arthritis also makes us use painkillers, some of which (NSAIDs) are bad for our arteries, kidneys, and blood pressure. So, any exercise that hurts your joints is bad for you and you should avoid it. After our thirties, and depending on our fitness level, we should be double careful about the type of exercises we do to burn calories, develop muscle, and stay healthy. Avoid joint injuries at all costs. A more moderate intensity exercise, like brisk walking, cycling, or swimming, may be a better choice for you.

Food and drinks

The type of food and drinks we put into our mouths can make or break our metabolisms. A diet rich in fruits, vegetables, and whole grains (the good carbs), with small quantities of good fats (olive oil, fish, unsalted nuts, avocado, and dark chocolate) and moderate amounts of lean protein (40–70 grams of protein a day is all that most of us need; for example, as much protein as there is in one-and-a-half chicken breasts or 8 glasses of milk) is a good diet. Such a diet promotes healthy metabolism and keeps our arteries clean. In contrast, a diet filled with bad carbs (cookies, desserts, donuts, milk chocolate, ice cream, candies, sugary soft drinks), trans and saturated fats (crispy baked goods like chips, red meat like beef and lamb, cold cuts, whole fat milk, and cheese) is a bad diet. Such a diet poisons our metabolisms and contributes to high cholesterol, belly fat, insulin resistance, type 2 diabetes, and high blood pressure. Eventually, a bad diet destroys our arteries by contributing to heart attacks and stroke. It is important to understand that every meal and every drink counts; daily consumption of healthy foods and unsweetened beverages helps keep our bellies free of fat, our metabolisms healthy, and our arteries clean. On the other hand, every unhealthy food and drink worsens our metabolisms and leads to microinjuries in our arteries. These microinjuries, when repeated day after day, contribute eventually to cholesterol plaques in the walls of our arteries that cannot be reversed. You need to understand that while mature cholesterol plaques can be later managed through healthy lifestyle and medications or even procedures, they cannot be undone; there is no human technology capable of removing cholesterol plaques and "cleaning" our arteries the same way that a dentist can clean the plaque from our teeth. In this respect, it is a pity we cannot directly see the insides of our arteries the same way we can look at our faces, skin, or our smiles in the mirror. As cholesterol plaques in the artery wall are invisible to us (unless specific medical imaging technology is used), we cannot directly see how ugly—let alone how dangerous—those cholesterol plaques look. Remember, heart attacks and strokes, although they strike suddenly, have been in the making for several decades. Every cookie, every donut, every cheeseburger moves us closer to unstable cholesterol plaques that can incite clots and cause heart attacks and stroke. It is important to understand, however, that even poison, in small quantities, does not kill. In other words, if you transgress a couple times a month, nothing bad will happen. It is the almost-daily bad diet habits that kill us.

Paleo and Mediterranean diets

Many diets claim important health benefits and weight loss but which one is the best for us? Which diet best provides us with the protein, vitamins, antioxidants, micronutrients, fiber, and energy that our bodies need to survive and prosper? I chose to briefly present two such popular diets, more to show the principles that should guide our food choices rather than strictly recommend the one or the other. These two diets are the:

- Paleo diet
- Mediterranean diet

The Paleo diet was popularized by Loren Cordain, Ph.D., Professor Emeritus, in the Department of Health and Exercise Science at Colorado State University and author of *The Paleo Diet*. The Paleo diet is based on fruits, vegetables, meats, eggs, seafood, nuts and seeds—foods that were likely consumed by our hunter-gatherer ancestors. As our genetic makeup has changed very little over the last 40,000 years, it makes sense to try to emulate the dietary patterns of the cavemen; our modern day human body was made to consume their type of food. It is important to note how different in quality were the meat and plants consumed by our ancestors compared to ours. Their meat was coming from game and free grazing animals; such a meat contained only 4% fat and was rich in healthful fats. The meat we buy today in the supermarket contains 25–30% fat and has much lower healthful fat content. Paleo diet is also rich in potassium and very low in sodium, the exact opposite of modern diet. Even the variety of Paleo fruits and vegetables is nutritionally different from ours; the plants that our ancestors used to eat had a higher protein to starch ratio than ours. One of the most important strengths of the Paleo diet is its low carb content; such a low carb content reduces the risk of metabolic disease like type 2 diabetes.

The Paleo diet excludes dairy products, grains, sugar, legumes, processed oils, salt, alcohol, and coffee. Some Paleo diet variants allow for an occasional glass of red wine. Some of the criticism against the Paleo diet includes that consumption of meat has been associated with heart disease, abnormal cholesterol, high blood pressure, and certain cancers. The Paleo counterargument is that the grain-fed beef and caged chickens of today have little resemblance to game, grass-fed animals, and free range chickens of the Paleo era. Another argument against Paleo is the proven health benefits of whole grains and legumes, foods that are excluded by Paleo diet.

The Mediterranean diet reflects the diet of the Mediterranean people (Greece, Southern Italy, Spain, and other countries in the Mediterranean basin) from the 1940s to early 1960 (as a more westernized diet was adopted in later years) . This diet was rich in extra virgin olive oil, whole grains, fruits, vegetables, and legumes. It also included dairy products, fish, and wine in moderate amounts. Red meat was consumed in only small quantities. Well-accepted health benefits of the Mediterranean diet include a reduction in heart and artery disease, type 2 diabetes, and cancer. This diet may also reduce the risk for Alzheimer's, although this is less well proven than its other health benefits. Another plus of the Mediterranean diet is that it is tasty, a factor that may help people stick with it in the long run.

Comparing the two diets, one can find both differences and similarities. The Paleo diet excludes grains, dairy and legumes, all elements of the Mediterranean diet. Whole grains and legumes have important health benefits. Whole grains reduce the risk of stroke, type 2 diabetes, artery and heart disease, and colon cancer. Legumes contain complex carbohydrates, protein, and fiber, and they help us feel fuller longer while they contain fewer calories than other high-satiety foods like fats or oils. Legumes also promote bowel regularity. Feta cheese, a typical Mediterranean diet dairy, has more water and less fat than popular types of cheeses like cheddar or swiss cheese. Both Paleo and the Mediterranean diets emphasize the need to stick to real food and avoid processed food; they both include fruits and vegetables, unsalted nuts, fish, and olive oil. The Mediterranean diet includes small amounts of meat, a moderate amount of eggs (including the yolk), and moderate amounts of alcohol, especially red wine.

Liver and pancreas

A healthy liver and pancreas are pillars of healthy metabolism. As you saw in Chapter 1, the liver is our key metabolic factory. The liver receives all the blood coming from the stomach and gut and, thus, it is the first stop for all digested and absorbed food. The liver transforms the foodstuff to "standard" format so that all the cells in the body can use it. The liver can make up cholesterol and sugar from scratch. It can also store sugar in the form of glycogen, make proteins, including cholesterol shuttles (LDL and HDL), reap the energy from fat, store vitamins and iron, and create bile, which is necessary for fat absorption. However, when we develop belly fat, the liver becomes "fatty liver" and is transformed to a factory of artery destruction. A "fatty liver" makes LDL models that are more dangerous than the usual LDL, as they are more capable of trespassing the artery lining (endothelium) and lodging into the artery wall where they start the buildup of cholesterol plaques. A fatty liver also creates a pro-inflammatory state and "insulin resistance," an environment where cells can no longer use sugar in a normal way. Insulin resistance contributes to high blood pressure and is a prelude to type 2 diabetes.

A healthy pancreas produces insulin, one of the most important hormones, as it regulates the metabolism of not only sugars but also fat and protein. In the face of belly fat, the pancreas, like the liver, becomes "fatty," with fat moving inside the pancreas and suffocating the beta cells that produce insulin. Therefore, belly fat is a "double whammy"; it creates both insulin resistance that strains the pancreas beta cells by demanding extra insulin production and, at the same time, destroys those beta cells. Eventually, beta cell demise leads to reduced insulin production and high blood sugar. This means prediabetes or type 2 diabetes.

Sleep

There is strong scientific evidence that sleeping less than seven hours a night is bad for our metabolisms. Stinting on sleep breeds insulin resistance, uninhibited food binges (almost exclusively bad carbs and bad fats), belly fat, and high blood pressure. Sleep deprivation increases the chance of one becoming diabetic; it also increases the risk of stroke by 33%.

How to build health wealth: invest in your metabolism to save your arteries

Creating and maintaining an environment of healthy metabolism (through near-daily practice of a healthy lifestyle) is the best way to support the health of our arteries in the long run. Such a health investment is like managing responsibly your finances, day after day, with your eyes not only on today but also on your future:

- "Live within your means and don't spend more than you make" translates into eat no more calories, through food and drinks, than those you can burn through motion and exercise.
- "Pay back your debt as soon as you can": lose these extra pounds of fat that make you obese or overweight and poison your metabolism as early in life as you can; the longer you wait, the more difficult the payback becomes.
- "Budgeting": know where your calories come from, how many they are, and how they are going to be burned; calories ingested but not used up will become belly fat and poison your metabolism.
- "Invest. Do things today for a more secure tomorrow": every day, find time for healthy activities that protect your future health, like preparing home meals using fresh ingredients, exercising, and sleeping for at least seven hours; also, make sure you build strong bones and muscle, know your numbers (e.g., blood pressure and LDL), and be current with immunizations and screening tests (see Chapter 5 for more details on healthy lifestyle).
- "Save for retirement": start a healthy lifestyle as early in life as you can in order to enjoy your retirement years.

Respect your health assets today, tomorrow, and in the long run

While almost no one (less than 3% of the adult US population) is perfectly healthy, preserving as many of our critical health assets as possible is the best health strategy we can afford. Consider that our biologic prime is around our mid twenties; after that we all start a slow decline that can be slowed down—if we consistently practice a healthy lifestyle—or accelerated—if we go for instant gratification, pleasure eating, and endless sitting. For this reason, the sooner we understand how our everyday actions impact our future health, the better. And as in saving for retirement, the earlier we start embracing wellness, the better; we preserve our valuable but vulnerable health assets for decades to come. Additionally, we have a responsibility, as adults, to be role models for the young, introduce them to healthy habits, and help them see the perils of an unhealthy lifestyle. It is important to understand that connecting an unhealthy behavior to a future consequence can be difficult for all of us, but it is even more difficult for our youngsters. According to Cindy Jardine, professor of Public Health at the University of Alberta, "...people aren't changing their behaviors, but it's not because they haven't gotten the information that these are big risks. We tend to sort of **live for now and into the limited future—not the long term**." So, help yourself and your kids see this "long term" and start your health savings now!

How to bring a healthy lifestyle into a busy daily schedule

Preparing healthy meals from scratch and creating opportunities for frequent physical activity are big challenges for today's busy person. In Chapter 7, I make the point that there are not enough hours in the day for most working Americans to incorporate a healthy lifestyle (including those seven to nine hours of sleep and two to four hours of physical activity) into their daily routine unless, as responsible members of the society in the era of obesity and diabetes, we find the resolve to drastically re-engineer the workplace and school (build structures and processes at work, at home, and at school that help us move our body more, eat healthy, sleep adequately, manage stress, and prevent obesity and diabetes. For example, we must take a strong position against addictive and dangerous (albeit tasty) added sugars. If the tobacco industry cannot advertise its products to minors, how come candies and sugary beverages are being advertised everywhere we look? We also need to ask ourselves why we are inviting kids to sit in the classroom (by providing classroom chairs) when they desperately lack movement and exercise.

For those who choose prevention and wellness early in life, the benefits are:
- A better health in the long run.
- Increased longevity by about 15 years.
- A better and more fulfilling life, with fewer medications and surgeries and less pain and disability.
- More independence, less Alzheimer's, and less need for nursing homes later in life.
- For those who want to to work till later in life, they can expect to perform as well as an individual 10 years younger.

Accept responsibility for your health

- **Information about our health is widely available; discuss it with your doctor, and this information may become knowledge.**

This is the internet era. Information about almost everything, including health matters, is widely available. Of course, you cannot believe everything you read in a random blog site; however, there are credible websites providing good information: WHO, NIH, CDC, the Mayo Clinic, and the Cleveland Clinic, just to mention a few. From these sites you get some basic idea about what health care concerns you may have (about you or a loved one), then you can discuss them with your doctor, and gradually this information becomes some basic knowledge. Then, you can take this basic knowledge about how you should live your life if you want to live long and stay in good health, apply it in your everyday life, and accept responsibility for your health. If disease strikes because you smoked, spent most your days sitting for 12 hours in front of a screen, or ate a ton of added sugars a day, you must accept that your choices contributed, at least in part, to your emphysema, your diabetes, or heart attack. Don't expect your doctors and other health care providers, hospitals, and clinics to always have a quick and easy solution, a magic bullet that will "fix" all your health problems and you will live happily ever after. This is too dangerous an illusion for any one of us to afford. An unhealthy lifestyle, along with aging and heredity, will almost certainly catch up with you at some point in time. As we have seen in previous chapters, added sugars, unhealthy fats, sitting and lack of physical activity, smoking, alcohol or drug abuse, or even stinting on sleep or working too many hours can have serious consequences for your health. Once your health is damaged, there are no easy, risk-free, inexpensive, or permanent treatments, even if provided by the best doctors and hospitals utilizing state-of-the-art technology and the most advanced procedures.

- **Even a perfect lifestyle will not prevent diseases of wear and tear or heredity.**

Additionally, even those who abide by a perfect lifestyle are subjected to the effects of aging and heredity, and these can bring serious disease later in life in spite of healthy living; a thin, physically active individual who has never smoked or eaten unhealthy may still develop high blood pressure or have high LDL cholesterol. If medications are not used, high blood pressure or LDL cholesterol will damage this person's arteries and can cause heart attacks, stroke, aneurysms, or even sudden death. These are basic medical facts that you must know.

- **Be the custodian of your own medical records.**

If you have ever had medical or surgical procedures and/or hospitalizations for important health conditions, it is very helpful that you keep records that can be available to any doctors you see in the future; you are the natural custodian of your own health records and should not relinquish this function to anybody else. Make it a habit to have an updated file of your most essential medical history and medication list. You have a very important and absolutely necessary role to play in protecting your health, preventing disease, and ensuring the best results when doctors or hospitals get involved in your care. These are no longer the times when the patient was expected to be a passive recipient of health care by doctors or nurses practicing in hospital or clinics. Today there is the internet, there are wearable fitness trackers, and your providers are much more open in educating you and answering your questions, to the best of their abilities (remember: doctors do not know everything). Your basic education in health matters is a necessity. For example, you are expected to know:

- What a healthy lifestyle is
- "Your Numbers" (e.g., blood pressure, waist circumference, blood sugar and A1c, LDL cholesterol and triglycerides and, ideally, hemoglobin, creatinine, and TSH)
- Your medications (and their dosage, as well as the reason why you are taking them) and allergies (if any)
- Your medical history and previous medical or surgical procedures

If you don't know any of these, ask your doctors, nurses, or other providers, and they will be happy to help you get there. But you need to want to get there and feel that this is your responsibility. If you feel insecure in obtaining and collecting this information, maybe another member in your family or a friend can help you and come with you in your doctor's appointments. But, please, do not accept a passive role in your care, thinking that the "the system" will take care of you. **Your health care starts with YOU!**

Your good health starts with you

Your good health depends heavily on keeping the health assets you got at your biologic prime (late teens for women, early twenties for men) for as long as possible. This is best achieved by:

- Not smoking
- Not abusing alcohol or drugs
- Being physically active almost every day while respecting your joints
- Eating right
- Sleeping well
- Avoiding accidents
- Managing stress
- Avoiding working third shift or more than 55 hours a week
- Being aware of side effects of over-the-counter medications
- Knowing your numbers (blood pressure, blood sugar, or A1c and cholesterol)
- Maintaining a good relationship with your primary care provider
- Seeking help when feeling unwell

Most of these things can be achieved by a knowledgeable YOU. Consider your primary care physician as your best health advisor and health coach and do not miss that annual wellness visit, even if you feel perfectly well or think you are too young to be sick. High blood pressure or high LDL do not cause any symptoms for years or decades while they are slowly destroying your arteries. Prediabetes or early diabetes can also be present with minimal or no symptoms. A dietician and a personal trainer can also provide valuable help in supporting your good health and maintaining your health assets.

So, do not be misled by any hospital or health insurance advertisement that wants you to believe you can live your life any way you want, being completely careless about your health and, in case you ever develop a heart attack or a stroke, a good hospital and insurance coverage will save you and give you back your health 100 percent. Would you be careless driving your car and allow yourself to get into a serious accident just because you have a good health insurance or there is a hospital with excellent trauma care close by? Without diminishing the huge significance of hospital treatment and good insurance coverage, these organizations are mostly providing "sick care" and "sick care" insurance, respectively (although the Affordable Care Act has required insurance plans to fully cover preventive services without copays or deductibles). Hospitals and doctors can treat but can rarely cure diseases. The suffering and disability a disease is causing cannot always be completely reversed. And even the best treatments (whether procedures or medications) can have side effects, many of them serious. **This is why there is nothing as valuable as disease prevention and wellness.** And remember, your good health starts with YOU and your health coaches: your primary care provider, a dietician, and a personal trainer.

More specifically, no hospital and no insurance can make your cholesterol plaques disappear from your arteries once they are there. What hospitals and good "health" insurance can do is fight for your life when the worst happens, when you are hit by a heart attack or a stroke, when you develop kidney failure or leg gangrene. They can minimize heart or brain damage, keep you alive in spite of kidneys that do not function, and they can save your leg or perform a successful leg amputation to save your life, provided you seek care as soon as possible after your symptoms begin and you are lucky. Notice the "fine prints" every time you sign a consent form prior to a medical or surgical procedure; read the list of potential complications that include serious health problems and even death and provide no guarantees. Do not have any illusions: if you do not fight for your health every day of your life, do not expect hospitals and health insurance companies to do it for you. **YOU** are your best health care; **YOU** are the one who holds most of the power to maintain your health assets. Your health care starts with you, with "a little help from your friends," your primary care physician and, when indicated, a dietician and a personal trainer.

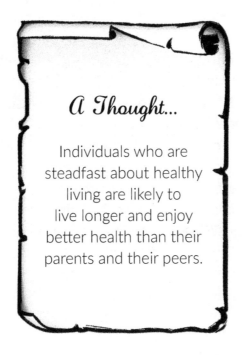

A Thought...

Individuals who are
steadfast about healthy
living are likely to
live longer and enjoy
better health than their
parents and their peers.

A consistently practiced healthy lifestyle will help us enjoy a family vacation when our friends (who smoked, ate, and sat incessantly) are undergoing open heart surgery or are recuperating from knee replacement surgery. "What we do for ourselves is often more important than what medicine can offer us" admits Harvard Medical School on its website "Harvard Health Publications."

So, how can you best preserve the health capital that was bestowed on you in your younger years? Is your chosen lifestyle a health asset or a liability?

These are some things that set apart the people who choose to live life the healthy way:

- Knowledge is power #1: they are educated about the perils of eating bad carbs and bad fats and of sitting the whole day; they are educated about prevention of obesity, diabetes, heart disease, stroke, cancer, depression, and Alzheimer's.
- Knowledge is power #2: they have learned the benefits of eating plenty of fruits and vegetables, small amounts of healthy fats (like olive oil, fish, and unsalted nuts), and adequate amounts of lean protein. They can tell whether a certain food is a health asset or liability.
- They put the effort #1: they prepare most of their meals using fresh ingredients at home.
- They put the effort #2: they exercise almost daily and may use wearable fitness trackers.
- They put the effort #3: at work they are not complacent but, instead, they grab every opportunity they can get to be physically active; they use standing desks, treadmill desks, or bicycle desks; they have a pair of dumbbells in their office and they frequently interrupt their sitting by standing up and moving around. Scientists suggest that simply standing up form our chair once every twenty minutes has important health benefits.
- They do not smoke.
- They monitor their body weight, waist circumference, and wear fitbits to count their daily steps; they also monitor their blood pressure at home.
- They have a good relationship with their primary care provider, and they know their numbers: their blood cholesterol (total, the bad LDL, the good HDL, and triglycerides), their blood sugar and A1c, and their blood pressure.
- They are aware of their family history, in particular whether any parent or sibling had type 2 diabetes, heart attack, stroke, bypass surgery, stents, or kidney failure.
- They sleep between seven and nine hours every night.
- If they drink alcohol, they never go overboard.

- They have some stress and they have learned how to best manage it. They also avoid situations that present them with excessive and lingering stress.
- They are happy with their work and family situation and set an example of healthy living for people around them.
- They have a purpose in life.
- Their social life is rich: they have friends and visit with them periodically, they have hobbies, they get out of the house frequently; and, if they retire, they have a structured schedule every day; they just don't sit around at home watching TV or purposelessly surfing the internet.

Limitations of medical treatment

One of the strongest arguments in favor of a healthy lifestyle in particular and disease prevention and wellness in general is that medicine, in spite of its remarkable progress, holds no fixes and no easy cures for diseases like obesity, diabetes, heart attacks, and stroke. Don't get me wrong: modern medicine, through medications and procedures, can abort a heart attack or a stroke and let the patient not only survive but also incur minimal losses of his heart or brain function. Through bariatric surgery it can reduce the weight of a 350 pound person by 150 pounds and, thus, relieve him or her of the need to take high blood pressure, diabetes, or cholesterol medications. But pay attention as to we doctors and other professionals approach the issue; we use the term disease "treatment," not disease cure. Modern medicine, in all its might, can provide exceptionally good treatment but not a cure.

But medical procedures have limitations, for example:
- Pills or surgical procedures for obesity are not a cure for obesity; when the pills stop, the weight is frequently gained back. Also, in spite of the tremendous weight loss from the several forms of bariatric surgery (Roux-en-Y gastric bypass surgery, gastric sleeve, or gastric ring), some of the weight lost is later regained. The most effective form of bariatric surgery (gastric bypass surgery) is also the most drastic one, necessitating vitamin supplementation for life and resulting in several lifelong symptoms.

- Heart bypass surgery does not fix the problem of cholesterol plaques in the heart arteries, as the grafts that "replace" our own arteries age and develop cholesterol plaques themselves within less than a decade after the operation (almost 10 percent of the grafts are already closed down by the time we leave the hospital).
- Heart bypass surgery is not equal to preventing the development of cholesterol blockages in the heart arteries in the first place. Heart arteries that are 50% clogged are likely to work better in the long run compared with brand new bypasses.
- Pills for high blood pressure or abnormal cholesterol are not equal to preventing high blood pressure or abnormal cholesterol in the first place. Once those pills are stopped, within a short period of time (a few days for the blood pressure and a few months for the blood cholesterol), blood pressure and abnormal cholesterol return to their previous morbid levels.
- Pills or insulin for diabetes do not cure diabetes. They simply lower blood sugar and reduce the chance of certain diabetic complications ("microvascular" complications like blindness, kidney failure, and nerve problems). Some of the pills as well as insulin, while directly lowering blood sugar, also lead to weight gain that can worsen diabetes. They can also lower blood sugar to unsafely low levels ("hypoglycemia").
- Preventing atrial fibrillation in the first place is much more preferable than developing it and either going through an ablation procedure to "cure" it (with its own risks and never 100 percent success rate) or taking medications to either prevent its recurrence (with the risk of several serious side effects) or prevent stroke, namely blood thinners (with their own set of complications).

In principle, medicine holds treatments for most diseases; these treatments favorably affect the pain, suffering, and threat to life posed by that disease but rarely, if ever, is medical treatment equally useful, simple, natural, and convenient as preventing the disease in the first place. No easy fixes!

Starting early in life

Best case scenario is to embrace wellness early in life. **How early is "early"?** It starts well before you are born and as soon as you are conceived. If your mother smokes, abuses alcohol, or does drugs, your life and health as a baby is already in grave danger. And being deprived of natural birth or breastfeeding does not allow the normal microorganisms to form in your bowel ("microbiome"). This may not sound too important, but it can certainly help you avoid asthma, allergies, infections, obesity, and heart disease later in your adult life. And, in your first few years in life, the diet your parents feed you, the physical activities they support you to perform, and the overall brain stimulation environment they build for you determines, in large part, how well you are going to do later in life, both physically and mentally. So, the burden for your healthy living early into your life falls more on the parents than on you. But, if you are a parent, consider that one of the best gifts you can give your child is, along with a brain-stimulating environment, a head start on a healthy way of life that will keep your child's belly fat to a minimum and his/her arteries and pancreas beta cells well protected.

Childhood

If you are a kid, these are the things your parents are supposed to guide (or make) you do:
- Play more with other children than you do with computers, game consoles, and smartphones.
- Avoid developing any belly fat. You have no excuse. You were born with a near-perfect body. You are not supposed to eat unhealthy meals just because it is convenient for your parents. Let your voice be heard! If you gain weight now, don't expect to shake it off later. Obese kids become obese adults.
- Getting used to eating fruits, vegetables, and legumes.
- Fast food and pizza should be an occasional transgression, not a habit.
- Eat at-home meals prepared from fresh ingredients.
- Avoid sugary beverages; ideally, tell your parents to not allow you to even taste them.
- Avoid prolonged sitting, at school and at home; learn to use standing and other non-sitting desks. Move or dance when watching videos. YouTube should not make "YouFat"!

- Know your numbers (or let your parents know them for you): your blood pressure, weight for height, blood sugar, cholesterol, HDL (the good cholesterol), LDL (the bad cholesterol), triglycerides. You see, nowadays even kids develop high blood pressure, high cholesterol, or type 2 diabetes. Should these diseases cross your path, please do not say "no" to medications just because it isn't "cool."

As is the case for all ages, for a healthy lifestyle to work, it needs to become a habit, and there is no better time than during your formative years. So, close your eyes and plunge into:
- Eating meals prepared at home from fresh ingredients
- Eating meals that are made of at least 50 percent fruits and vegetables
- Being physically active for several hours a day

Eating healthy and moving around should come natural to you, without even the need to use your brain; it should be your default mode unless something more important needs your attention, like homework. Still, you can use a standing desk.

The pressure from the obesity-diabetes-artery disease epidemic is so acute that I can argue that learning and experiencing healthy lifestyle at school is more important than the school curriculum itself. Obese and overweight kids become diabetic adults. This is certainly not the future we plan for our children. Healthy experiences for school-age children can include:
- Chairless classrooms.
- Peripatetic teaching sessions—the way one walks around in a museum while the guide is pointing to the exhibits. Walking classrooms are already happening in the US.
- A science curriculum built around the biology of obesity, diabetes, and artery disease. The epidemic provides us with rich material helpful not only to the kids themselves but also to their parents.

As childhood obesity rates have tripled since the 1970s and kids get diagnosed with high blood pressure and type 2 diabetes (almost unheard of 40 years ago, being almost exclusively adult-only diseases), how should their parents respond? Parents, think of what belly fat does to your child's liver and pancreas. Once these pancreas beta cells are stifled by local fat and insulin resistance (a result of belly fat and fatty liver, that is junk food and endless hours sitting in front of the computer or TV), these beta cells are gone and are not coming back, no matter what. The result? Type 2 diabetes for the rest of your kid's life. And the longer one lives with diabetes, the more likely he or she is to suffer its complications, like heart attacks, stroke, blindness, kidney failure, or leg amputations. Don't you want to steer your kid clear of all this trauma?

Unhealthy diet and playing too many computer games destroys the lining of your kids' young arteries; once LDL passes through this lining, it creates "fatty streaks," the earliest stage of cholesterol plaque development. Once these cholesterol plaques call the artery wall their home, there is no technology in the world that can get them out of there and "clean your arteries out."

Parents, do the best you can to protect your child's arteries! Your kids (and teenagers) are never going to have the luxury of such a busy and robust metabolism!

As an adolescent

As rates of childhood obesity have soared and metabolic diseases are now diagnosed in kids, many adolescents find themselves already in metabolic trouble: abdominal obesity, high blood pressure, high cholesterol, or even diabetes. What led them there?
- Screenplay instead of real play
- Chicken nuggets instead of fruits and vegetables
- Fast food meals and sugary beverages instead of home meals and water

No matter what the reason, it is a sad truth that some of our adolescents have already amassed fat in their bellies and developed insulin resistance, pancreatic beta cell demise, and fatty livers, hence the high cholesterol, high blood pressure, and diabetes. That's a tough cardiometabolic "endowment" for the rest of these youngsters' lives.

To avoid this mess so early in life, parents need to be steadfast and lead with the way to healthy habits for their offspring with authority. Additionally, age-appropriate educational material can help adolescents see for themselves the big mess they are getting into if they make the wrong lifestyle choices early in life. **Obesity and its complications are not cool!**

Here is some advice for our teenagers with emphasis on cardiometabolic health:

- Stay physically active; be involved in sports but avoid injuries.
- Don't pick up smoking.
- Don't start alcohol or drugs.
- Avoid becoming fat; if you are obese, try to lose weight. Your best chance for losing weight is during your teenage years, as your metabolism is at its prime, your joints are healthy, and your muscles strong so you can move without pain and lose this weight. These opportunities for burning calories that easily won't come again in your life!
- Eat fruits, vegetables, and legumes daily; this is the time to pick up healthy eating habits.
- Use low-fat dairy products and lean proteins.
- Eat meals prepared at home and with fresh ingredients.
- Avoid sugary beverages.
- Avoid prolonged sitting and, instead, commit to non-sitting arrangements at school and at home. Learn to use standing desks.
- Know your numbers: blood pressure, weight for height, blood sugar, cholesterol, HDL (the good cholesterol), LDL (the bad cholesterol), and triglycerides.
- Be educated about diseases that threaten you at your age range, including obesity, type 2 diabetes, high blood pressure, high cholesterol, and artery disease.

And while it has very little to do with protecting your arteries from cholesterol plaque, the following advice has a lot to do about preserving your life. So, according to CDC:

Be aware that driving between the ages of 16 and 19 is three times as risky as driving at age 20 or older. Be extremely cautious in your early driving years and avoid driving at night. A car driven by a teenager with teen passengers is a very risky proposition. Never text or drink and drive or drive under the influence of drugs; observe traffic signs and speed limits.

In your twenties and thirties

This is the first time in your life that YOU are calling the shots! It is also probably the first time that you see in practice that rights come hand in hand with responsibilities:

- You have the right to play and the responsibility to pay (and I don't just mean "money").
- You have the right to choose your job and the responsibility to abide by the time and activity commitments it demands and to live within the means of the income that it provides.
- You have the right to choose your spouse and the responsibility to compromise and stay together, especially if you have children.
- You have the right to eat donuts and bacon every day and the responsibility to have a pretty good health and life insurance.
- You have the right to sit in front of a computer twelve hours a day and the responsibility to take care of your high blood pressure, hurting knees, or diabetes.

So, the time for blaming "others" is over. Yours are the successes and the failures. And since you may also be starting a family of your own and have kids, it is important to show leadership in guiding your children not only towards what is "cool" but also to what is healthy and right. Set the right example for your loved ones; you are no longer by yourself. Help those around you learn early in their life about the risks of obesity, diabetes, heart and artery disease, of sitting for too long and not eating fruits and vegetables. Once your healthy lifestyle has become a fun habit for you, it can also become a great example for the people around you.

The key health objective for this stage in your life is **maintaining as many of your health assets as possible**, like:

- Well-developed muscles that can sustain a healthy metabolism.

- Healthy joints that allow you to use your muscles without causing pain.
- Robust pancreas beta cells capable of producing necessary amounts of insulin.
- Arteries with as few cholesterol plaques as possible.
- Flexible (not just strong) heart muscle. Stiffening of the heart muscle (diastolic dysfunction) is common after the age of 35 and can cause shortness of breath; it can also cause serious problems later in life, like heart failure and atrial fibrillation).

How do you know you are on the right path?

- You don't smoke (cigarettes or anything else).
- You have no belly fat (fat under your belly's skin does not count as belly fat; belly fat—unhealthy fat—is only the fat deep in your abdomen; this fat is a sign of an unhealthy metabolism and a red flag for your arteries. If your waist circumference is above 38 inches for men or 33 inches for women, you have at least some belly fat.
- Your blood pressure is below 120/80 mmHg.
- Your LDL is below 130 mg/dl.
- Your fasting blood sugar is below 100 mg/dl, and your A1c is below 5.7%.
- You can climb up two flights of stairs without any shortness of breath.
- You don't abuse alcohol (do not drink more than two drinks a day for men or one drink a day for women).
- You don't use drugs.
- You sleep at least seven hours per night and you avoid working third shift.
- Every day you do at least 15,000 steps.
- You sit for less than six hours a day.

But these are not always easy things to achieve. What if you are failing in some of these areas?

- If you smoke, you may be on the path of developing emphysema in your fifties and heart attacks in your late thirties or forties, although not every smoker does. Smoking can negate all other good healthy behaviors.

- If you do have some belly fat (waist circumference above 38 inches for men or 33 inches for women), you can assume that there is also fat in your liver ("fatty liver," meaning insulin resistance), in your pancreas (increasing the risk of becoming diabetic), in between your muscles (another contributor of insulin resistance), or inside your heart muscle (predisposing you to develop heart stiffness and diastolic dysfunction).
- A blood pressure between 120–139/80–89 is a step forward to high blood pressure called "prehypertension" and a warning sign of developing true high blood pressure.
- If your blood pressure is 140/90 or higher, you do have high blood pressure ("hypertension"). If abandoning salt and fast and processed foods, losing weight, and exercising do not lower your blood pressure to normal levels, you will need to start medications or permanent problems with your heart, arteries, and kidneys may be just a few years away.
- In case your LDL is above 130 mg/dl, you need to keep a close eye on it, with the help of your health care provider. Unless you have already developed artery disease or diabetes, high blood pressure, or have a parent or a sibling with heart attacks at a young age, or are a smoker, or your LDL is at least 190, you don't need medications. Stick to a healthy diet and lots of physical activities and follow the advice of your family doctor.
- If your (fasting) blood sugar is between 100–125 or your A1c between 5.7 and 6.5%, you are prediabetic. That means you are at higher risk of becoming diabetic over the next 5–10 years, especially if there is type 2 diabetes in your immediate family (parent or sibling) and have even small amounts of belly fat.
- If your fasting blood sugar is 126 or higher or A1c is 6.5% or higher, you are diabetic. If diet and exercise don't help you move out of the diabetic range, you need to start medications. Diabetes diagnosis is not a death sentence, but it is serious and is a definite milestone in your life. You will no longer be allowed to eat carbs the way you used to. You are likely to need daily medications and self monitoring of your blood sugar by pricking your finger. You are also placed at a

high-risk category for developing artery disease and other serious complications (like kidney failure or blindness) in the future. Diabetes grants you a grace period of five to seven years, but being too cozy about your blood sugar control will almost guarantee serious trouble in the future. If you are a diabetic who smokes, your risk for artery disease is so high that heart attacks, stroke, belly aneurysm, or clogged leg arteries become only a matter of time.

- If you get out of breath easily, please be checked by your doctor. Although it may just be that you are no longer as fit as you used to be or that you are overweight, shortness of breath can be a symptom of serious heart or lung disease.
- If you abuse alcohol and drugs, please seek help. Continuing to do so can ruin your health, your job, your finances, and the life of the people around you.
- Stinting on sleep, working third shift, and working longer than 55 hours a week are all bad for your health. While the consequences are not immediate, you don't want inadequate sleeping or an unbalanced life-work schedule to make your body look and feel 10 years older than your birth date suggests.
- Inadequate physical activity and/or prolonged sitting are a prelude to obesity, diabetes, high blood pressure, and abnormal cholesterol.

So, these are the things you need to do:
- Stay physically active; do a combination of exercises: cardio (aerobic), strengthening, stretching, and balancing; avoid injuries.
- Be physically active at work and at home for a minimum of two hours every day.
- Avoid heavy weight lifting and straining, as this type of exercise (isometric with straining and holding your breath) can raise your blood pressure to unsafe levels and destroy your heart and your aorta.
- Don't pick up smoking; if you smoke, quit.
- Use alcohol in moderation.
- Do not use drugs.
- If you have abdominal obesity, try to lose weight. If you cannot lose weight, try very hard to not add even a single pound of fat to your belly.

- Sleep between seven and nine hours every night.
- Try to avoid employment that forces you to work more than 55 hours per week or work third shift; you may need the money, but it is a bad investment for your health.
- Know your numbers: blood pressure, waist circumference, blood sugar and A1c, cholesterol, HDL (the good cholesterol), LDL (the bad cholesterol), and triglycerides.
- Educate yourself about obesity, type 2 diabetes, high blood pressure, high cholesterol, and artery disease.
- Is either of your parents or any siblings type 2 diabetic? If so, place even more emphasis on staying physically active for more than two hours a day. Eat fresh fruits and vegetables and limit animal fat and salt.
- Avoid chronic use of certain medications like NSAIDs (available over the counter under the names ibuprofen, naproxen and diclofenac and a large number of brand names), as they can cause kidney failure, heart attacks, heart failure, high blood pressure, high potassium, stomach irritation, and bleeding complications.
- Avoid chronic use of opioids (codeine, hydrocodone, methadone, morphine, fentanyl), as they double the risk of heart attacks, possibly through abnormal sleep patterns.
- If you are overweight or obese, snore at night, and have high blood pressure, get checked for sleep apnea, a common and dangerous condition that can be helped without the use of medications.
- If you are severely obese (BMI above 40) and have developed type 2 diabetes, high blood pressure, or sleep apnea, you may want to consider weight-loss ("bariatric") surgery. This may reverse diabetes or other obesity-related diseases.

Also be aware that, as we move from our late teens/early twenties to our midlife years, important changes happen to our body, even if our lifestyle remains perfectly healthy. As we pass our biological prime (late teens for women, early twenties for men) if we are not careful and disciplined, we may start losing our biologic assets in a hurry:

- Belly fat breeds abnormal metabolism, fatty liver, insulin resistance, fatty pancreas, muscle weakening, and heart stiffening (diastolic dysfunction).

- Belly fat at age 30-plus also means that you can no longer eat as much salt as you want. Your kidneys are more likely to retain it, and this may lead to high blood pressure early in life, especially if you have a family history of high blood pressure.
- Abnormal metabolism and insulin resistance bring high blood pressure and cholesterol, prediabetes and diabetes, and, finally, artery disease like heart attacks and stroke. It takes a few decades to get there, as your youth is still somewhat protecting you.
- Smoking and abuse of alcohol and drugs are other ways that eat away your health assets, one cigarette, one drink, one joint, one day at a time.
- Careless driving and aggressive overall behavior can hurt your physical and emotional health in many ways, even if your arteries escape damage.

A healthy lifestyle can keep your health assets you are endowed with at your biological prime as intact as possible for many decades to come. Your health assets are even more valuable and irreplaceable than your financial assets, but once they are depreciated, their lost value can never be recovered. So, respect and preserve your health endowment.

In your forties and fifties

Hello middle age!

Are you going to greet middle age with a lean and robust body or, like most of your peers, with a plump belly? Belly fat becomes so common in our forties and fifties, even for individuals who do take good care of their health. As we discussed before, abdominal obesity means also fatty liver, fatty pancreas, fatty muscle, and fatty heart, meaning you are on your way towards:

- Insulin resistance
- High blood pressure
- Abnormal cholesterol
- Prediabetes or diabetes
- Artery disease (heart attacks, stroke, sudden death, clogging of the leg arteries)

At the same time, along with some belly fat, middle age introduces us to new realities, like some degree of arthritis in the knees, hips, back, and hands. At this point, strenuous exercise routines may further hurt our joints. Painful joints are a far-reaching problem, as they:

- Force us to use our muscle less because it hurts; less muscle use means slower metabolism and higher chances for artery disease.
- May force us to take certain painkillers (like NSAIDs or opioids) that, by themselves, can have grave health consequences (NSAIDs threaten our heart and kidneys, and opioids can cause addiction and central sleep apnea).

So, as it's true for the 20 and 30 year olds, **maintaining as many of your health assets as possible** continues to be a key health objective. By our forties and fifties, though, some wear and tear is inevitable and even a healthy lifestyle cannot fully prevent a small health asset depreciation. The ultimate fear is artery disease, like heart attacks and stroke. But while our arteries are "out of sight," they should not be "out of mind." We need to be aggressive in managing any and all undepreciated and undamaged health assets we still posses:

- If abdobese or insulin resistant, put even more emphasis on healthy eating and adequate physical activity to maintain a level of metabolism not much lower than you did in your twenties and thirties. Minimum of 15,000 steps a day, light weights, at least every other day, lots of fruits, vegetables, and whole grains, and rare diet transgressions.
- If, in spite of your best health efforts, you have already developed high blood pressure, high cholesterol, prediabetes, or diabetes, discuss with your doctor about the need to start taking medications. I know that you will hate this; I hear it all the time from my patients. No one wants side effects, like dizziness, reduced sexual drive, or muscle aches. But what about the "side effects" of high blood pressure, high cholesterol, or diabetes? Keep in mind that **every day you spend with high blood pressure, high LDL cholesterol, or undertreated diabetes means a microdamage to your arteries that will never go away.** And when time comes, those accumulated artery microdamages will sweep around your system like a tornado,

leaving a path of destruction that modern medicine may not have the technology to undo and rebuild.

As a 40 to 50 year old, how do you know you are on the right path-healthwise?

- You don't smoke (cigarettes or anything else).
- You have no or minimal belly fat.
- Your blood pressure is below 120/80 mmHg.
- Your LDL is below 130 mg/dl.
- Your fasting blood sugar is below 100 mg/dl and A1c below 5.7%.
- You can climb up two flight of stairs without any shortness of breath.
- You don't abuse alcohol (do not drink more than two drinks a day for men or one drink a day for women).
- You don't use drugs.
- You sleep at least seven hours per night and you avoid working third shift.
- Every day you do at least 15,000 steps.
- You sit for less than six hours a day.
- You have a sincere partnership/relationship with your primary care provider; between the two of you, you know your numbers (waist circumference, blood pressure, LDL, triglycerides, blood sugar, A1c), and you stay current on acceptable screening tests and immunizations.

Some other points to consider in your forties and fifties:

- Joint cartilage does not regenerate.
- Muscle mass is declining.
- Our bodies do not handle sodium (salt) well, linking high salt consumption to higher blood pressure.
- Our main arteries and heart muscle lose their elasticity, leading to higher BP and stiffening of the heart (diastolic dysfunction), respectively. These changes set the stage for the future development of advanced heart and artery disease, like atrial fibrillation, diastolic heart failure, heart attacks, and stroke.

- Knowing your health numbers—blood pressure, waist circumference, blood sugar and A1c, cholesterol, HDL, LDL, and triglycerides— is even more important in midlife, as many of us have already developed high blood pressure, prediabetes, diabetes, or abnormal cholesterol that may have gone undiagnosed.
- Many of us diagnosed with high blood pressure or very high LDL cholesterol refuse to take medications. The argument goes like this: how come I need to take medications with serious side effects when I feel and look well? The answer is that you can't see your arteries; you're using the "out of sight, out of mind" reasoning to kid yourself that all is well. Do you know what the "side effects" of high blood pressure and high LDL on your arteries are? Do you know that the everyday microdamages to your arteries will never go away?
- Among the most difficult patients to persuade to take blood pressure or cholesterol medications are those who abide by a healthy lifestyle: they do not smoke, they exercise almost daily, they eat healthy, they do not abuse alcohol, and their weight and waist circumference are normal. These individuals, while commendable for their achievements, ignore that biology is what it is; it knows no fairness. Yes, it will reward a healthy lifestyle, but not always in absolute terms. Thus, you may be a marathon runner with the body of an adolescent and live an impeccable lifestyle and, yet, your blood pressure or bad cholesterol (LDL)—in part due to genetics and in part due to aging—may be through the roof.
- "Natural" remedies may help a slightly elevated blood pressure or cholesterol (garlic, for example, can lower the blood pressure by about 3 mmHg, and fish oil supplements will lower triglycerides to some extent). If your blood pressure is 180/100 (mmHg) or your LDL above 190 (mg/dl), don't expect much help from "natural" remedies or herbs. The effect of high blood pressure or high LDL on the arteries is going to be similar whether you are obese and sedentary or thin and athletic, whether you live on fast food or you are a vegetarian.
- Patients with diabetes are less likely than those with high blood pressure or high LDL to refuse medications. Diabetes usually causes symptoms, like increased thirst and urination and unexplained weight loss. Also, in popular culture, diabetes looms as a bigger

threat to our health and is taken more seriously than high blood pressure or high LDL. As a result, it is much easier to persuade a diabetic patient to start taking medications for his or her blood sugar.

In your sixties and beyond

You have made it! And while aging is not for wimps, think of how many of your friends and colleagues were never given the opportunity to experience what life has to offer in this stage, like:

- The unmatched and fun human experience of being around your grandchildren
- The opportunity to have more time for yourself, family, and loved ones
- A chance to become a volunteer
- A unique perspective on life, based on the wisdom and maturity you have accumulated over the years
- Learning a new language or a musical instrument, reading books, studying history and religion
- Traveling
- In case you want to keep working, the experience of serving at a senior position, using your maturity and complex reasoning and social skills
- A sense of accomplishment

The ways our bodies change from our forties to our mid-sixties and beyond

Even for those who lived as healthy a lifestyle as possible, a healthy 60 is not like a healthy 20; we have to contend ourselves with new realities, and this goes beyond wrinkles and gray hair. Due to aging (both programmed in our genes and as a result of wear-and-tear), our muscles, beta pancreatic cells, arteries, and joints change dramatically. Our kidneys, eyes, ears, and skin also show conspicuous changes.

- As we age, we lose muscle. This is called "sarcopenia of aging" and starts in our thirties and forties but becomes accelerated after our mid fifties. Working out at least every other day with light or moderate weights helps cancel or even reverse this muscle loss.

- Our beta pancreatic cells produce insulin, a vital hormone for our metabolism. As a result of belly fat (which also implies fat inside the pancreas), heredity (a parent or a sibling with type 2 diabetes), and aging, the ability of beta cells to produce insulin is reduced over time. Insulin resistance (abdominal obesity and fatty liver) might have been demanding a higher production rate from our beta cells ever since we developed belly fat. The two processes work together to exhaust and kill our beta cells. When beta cell ability to produce insulin falls below a certain level, we become diabetic.

- Even a healthy lifestyle cannot entirely prevent cholesterol plaques from forming in the walls of our arteries later in life. A healthy lifestyle (and a bit of good luck), though, can help prevent heart attacks before our seventies or eighties.

- Joint cartilage stops regenerating after our body has stopped growing (late teens/early twenties). Although some cartilage damage occurs even if we take care of our joints, the excessive wear and tear associated with obesity and sports injuries may leave us with arthritic joints as early as in our late twenties. By the time we reach our sixties, some arthritis is common not only in our knees but also in our hands, hips, back, and shoulders. This does not mean, however, that all of us will require joint replacement surgery or daily NSAIDs or opioids. Good joint functionality can remain in spite of some level of arthritis.

- Kidney function declines as we age. This decline is faster if we develop diabetes, high blood pressure, artery disease, or obesity or if we frequently use certain medications (primarily NSAIDs). If we escape diabetes and keep blood pressure controlled with lifestyle and medications (even if we are diagnosed with high blood pressure), we can expect a long life without major kidney problems.

- Beyond the need for eyeglasses sometime in our forties, aging can contribute to macular degeneration, cataracts, glaucoma, and dry eye. Eye disease is an important "microvascular" complication of diabetes and is worse the higher our A1c is above 6.5–7.0%. CDC suggests that "everyone age 50 or older should visit an eye care professional for a comprehensive dilated eye exam."

- A combination of declining hearing acuity and a poor eyesight can lead not only to social isolation and increased accidents but has also been associated with increased heart and artery disease mortality, especially in older men.
- An unhealthy lifestyle (smoking, poor diet, obesity, alcohol, or drug abuse) and heredity, as well as sun exposure make our skin prone to damage. The skin loses elasticity, forming wrinkles; it may also develop cancer.

In case we neglected our health earlier in life (through bad diet, sedentary lifestyle, development of belly fat, untreated high blood pressure or LDL cholesterol, smoking, abusing alcohol or drugs), the damage our organs will have suffered by the time we reach our sixties will be significant and largely irreversible. Slow metabolism, loss of functionality, pain, and other symptoms, and artery complications (heart attacks and stroke) are to be expected. By sticking to prevention and wellness as early in life as possible and keeping a will-not-let-go attitude later in life, we concede only the absolute minimum to the aging process and we keep a good metabolism, good functionality, and minimal symptoms till our very late years in life. Monitoring our health also allows us to discover artery and heart disease early and increases our chances of successful treatment.

Health priorities in our sixties and beyond:

- Opt for functionality, even if your health is not perfect. For example, you may still be able to play sports and travel in spite of arthritis, learn new things in spite of memory lapses, and prevent heart attacks, heart failure, atrial fibrillation, and stroke in spite of high blood pressure, high cholesterol, prediabetes, or diabetes.
- Avoid or manage obesity; counteract obesity with a couple of hours of moderate physical activity every day, including all three forms of exercise (cardio, strengthening, and stretching/balance).
- Don't smoke.
- Don't abuse alcohol.
- Stay physically active.
- Eat a healthy diet rich in fruits, vegetables, and whole grains.
- Keep a rich social life.

- Have a structured daily schedule even after your retirement; don't stay at home the entire day sitting in front of a TV or a computer screen.
- Have a strong reason to want to live; absence of purpose in this age range can lead into depression and quick dwindling of our physical health.
- Have a close relationship with your primary care doctor based on good chemistry, mutual trust, and respect.
- Monitor your health. You monitor your financial situation. Doesn't your health deserve the same? At least once a week, monitor your blood pressure and pulse rate, your waist circumference and body weight, and the number of steps you walk. The future may bring wearable technologies that will allow you to monitor with great degree of accuracy many more important things (like your blood sugar and the quality of your sleep, for example).
- Keep your essential medical records (major diagnoses, medications, procedures, and test results) in a file. Taking these records with you to every doctor you see for a first time will make your care smooth and effective. In this way you will be helping your doctor help you best.
- Take any medications you are on for high blood pressure, high cholesterol, or any other chronic diseases to your appointment with your physician.
- Learn from your doctor what medications' side effects to watch for. Using the internet to learn about medication side effects is not a good idea, as the few common side effects are lost in a sea of hundreds of uncommon or uncertain side effects. Pharmaceutical companies are obligated by law to test their drugs for the possibility of side effects in a large number of individuals. They are obligated to report anything that these individuals are complaining of as side effects, even if not caused by the drug. For example, if a person who took the drug feels dizzy for a reason totally unrelated to the drug, the pharmaceutical company has to mention 'dizziness' as a side effect of this drug. Imagine that you search the internet about the side effect profile of a medication and you find a list of 300 such side effects. Which one are real and which are not? Try it for yourself: write down a list of any symptoms you can imagine and

then look up the side effects of your medicines on the internet. Then compare the two lists!

- Be educated about your health and your own health problems and maintain a strong and productive relationship with your primary care provider.
- Stay current with screening tests (for colon, breast, and prostate cancer, for example) and immunizations.

Chapter 4 Questions

1. Which of the following supports a healthy metabolism?
   - Drinking one alcoholic beverage a day
   - Smoking two cigarettes a day
   - Sitting 10 hours a day
   - Sleeping five hours a day

2. Name four foods that contain healthy fats.
   - a.
   - b.
   - c.
   - d.

3. Which of the following is a worse metabolic sign?
   - A blood pressure of 130/82 mmHg
   - An A1c of 8%
   - Triglycerides of 150 mg/dl
   - Waist circumference of 40 inches on a white male

4. What is better for the metabolism of a healthy 40-year-old man?
   - Two 12-ounce beers every day
   - Six 12-ounce beers on Friday and Saturday only

5. What causes more people to die in Western countries?
   - High LDL cholesterol
   - Side effects of statins

6. Which is a better blood pressure for a 30-year old woman?
   - 98/70 mmHg
   - 132/70 mmHg
   - 110/86 mmHg
   - 140/90 mmHg

7. Who is the best custodian of your personal health records?
   - Your primary care provider

- Your heart specialist
- The hospital where you had a gallbladder surgery and a stress test
- You
- The government

8. Who has more body muscle?
   - A 30-year old construction worker
   - A 70-year old retired marathon runner
   - A 22-year old healthy female

Chapter 5

THE PATH DOWN THE MIDDLE
OF THE ROAD

"Those who think they have no time for exercise will sooner or later have to find time for illness."
—Edward Stanley

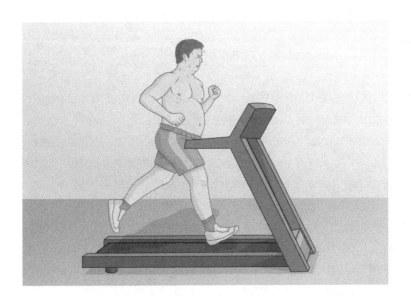

Some of us eat healthy, exercise daily, have very little or no belly fat, and do not smoke. Others are obese and smokers and they could care less about becoming diabetic or developing heart disease. There is no way to persuade them to quit their cigarettes, their burgers, or their six packs of beer. This is the path they have chosen in life, and they are not going to listen to anyone who tries to talk health sense to them.

And then, there is most of us: those in the middle. Not entirely "allergic" to fruits and vegetables and not complete foreigners to the gym or the home treadmill. We do not always lend a deaf ear to calls for giving up fast food, reducing red meat and sugary drinks, cutting back on cookies and ice cream. However, healthy eating or daily exercising is not exactly our "passion." We do visit our health care providers (sometimes), and we are frequently on top of our mammograms, pap smears, colonoscopies, and flu shots. We do have some degree of belly fat, and some of us are current or former smokers. Some of us binge on alcohol or smoke an occasional joint. Blood pressure and LDL cholesterol might have been issues but, at least occasionally, we remember to take our medicines.

And many of us are happy the way we are. We feel that we are perfectly well balanced between the two extremes: those health fanatics who miss out on life's enjoyment and those who show complete disrespect for their lives and health and die suddenly of a heart attack in their forties or have a stroke and are left paralyzed in their fifties. If we, occasionally, get some shortness of breath, knee pains (an ibuprofen a day will keep the pain away), low back pain (an oxycontin from time to time), or sleep apnea (we do use our sleep mask), it is not the end of the world; we will put up with it. If you warn us that our blood sugar is in the prediabetes range (and our mother was a diabetic) and that our risk of stroke, heart attacks, and heart failure is high, we will listen. But man, do not expect us to let go of every bit of joy life has to offer just to live a few more years. After all, we are all going to die someday. And if you try to scare us about a "high risk of heart attack," dying suddenly in our sleep may be the best way to go. But not in our fifties!

Those in the middle of the road, that is those individuals whose attitude regarding physical activity, diet, smoking and alcohol use falls squarely in the middle between healthy and unhealthy lifestyle as well as those who, in spite of a clearly unhealthy lifestyle, want to improve their health, make up the most of us. They are the most promising target of the campaign to defeat the obesity-diabetes-artery disease epidemic. These are the people that need to be supported in their efforts to improve their lifestyles; that's how we can turn the tide of this epidemic. And here is why:

- Those in the middle are the majority. They probably make up at least 50 percent of all American adults.
- They are, to a certain extent, willing to both listen and act accordingly to improve their lifestyles.
- Many of those in the middle of the road have not yet tried to change their lifestyles because they are intimidated by strict diet or exercise requirements and they are afraid of failure.

How can we estimate how many they are?

We can only get an approximated idea, a rough estimate of how many those in the middle of the road are. Precise figures are almost impossible to obtain for several reasons:

Like most things in medicine, there is no crisp dividing line separating healthy from unhealthy eating, sedentary from active lifestyle, smoking from not smoking, and healthy versus unhealthy alcohol use. Consider the following questions:

- If you eat more than five portions of fruits and vegetables every day (a healthy habit) but you also eat steak 5 times a week (an unhealthy habit), is your diet healthy or unhealthy?
- You do walk 30 minutes a day, five days a week as the recommendations for minimum physical activity for American adults call for. But you also sit in front of a computer 12 hours a day, a very unhealthy habit. Do you score high or low in the physical activity domain?
- You used to smoke half a pack a day but quit three days ago; or you have been a "light" smoker, smoking only two to three cigarettes a day, are you a smoker or not? Scientific data argue that you are still a smoker, as it takes between three to five years of abstinence from smoking to lower your risk for heart attacks to the level of the

non-smoker. Don't forget that even two cigarettes a day are plenty capable of causing a heart attack.

- You drink beer only twice a week. During the weekends you get together with your friends and drink four to six beers at a time. Your daily average is less than two alcoholic drinks per day (healthy alcohol consumption is defined as one or two alcoholic beverages a day for men younger than 65 years or one drink a day for women or men 65 years and older), but you are a binge drinker. Is this bad for your health?
- You smoke and eat an unhealthy diet. But you truly want to change. You are serious about quitting smoking and starting eating healthy. Shouldn't you be counted as a middle of the road based on your aspirations?

This brings us to a very important question: Do we know how many among us are in "the middle of the road"? While it is almost impossible to know the exact number, they are probably the majority. And here is why:

Data from the US Department of Health and Human services suggest, for example, that three out of four Americans do not eat the recommended minimum five portions of fruits and vegetables a day, that 70% eat more saturated fat and added sugars than the recommended amount, and 85% consume more salt than what is considered healthy. Also, between 16 and 18 percent of the population are smokers.

A very interesting study published in Mayo Clinic Proceedings in 2016 by Loprinzi et al. found that **less than 3 percent of all Americans are currently practicing a healthy lifestyle** and have ideal amounts of body fat. While we would expect that those of us who are doing everything right are a minority, 3 percent is an astonishing and unexpectedly low figure. Looking a bit closer at the data though, we see that, for the purpose of this study, in order to be counted as having a perfect lifestyle you should:

- have never been a smoker
- exercise almost daily
- eat a perfectly healthy diet

On top of that, your body fat should be low. Body fat is, however, the result of lifestyle (not part of the lifestyle itself) and is influenced by so many other factors than diet and exercise, including heredity, age, race, ethnic background, whether you breastfed as a baby, whether you were born through natural birth, and what kind of diet you consumed as a baby; these factors have very little to do with whether your current behavior and chosen lifestyle is healthy or unhealthy, thus the 3 percent figure looks unrealistically low. Still, by combining all the data from this and other studies, it appears that no more than 10–15 percent of American adults score high in all the lifestyle areas (their diet is healthy and they exercise almost daily and they are non-smokers). The same data suggests that between 10 and 30 percent of American adults are doing all the wrong things in regards to their lifestyle: they smoke and eat unhealthy and do not perform the recommended amount of physical activity. So we are left with about 60 to 70 percent of American adults that seem to be exactly in the middle of the road. As this percentage represents the majority, chances are that you and me and most of our loved ones, friends, colleagues, and other acquaintances fall into this category: the middle of the road!

So, let's examine the attitudes of those middle-of-the-road people in regards to improving their lifestyles.

While some are happy the way they are, many realize what is at stake and are willing to change. They see some of their friends and relatives getting heart attacks in their forties, open heart surgeries and diabetes in their fifties, strokes in their sixties, and they don't like it. They turn to themselves, sometimes after the "encouragement" of their spouse. They don't like their fat belly, their shortness of breath, their cigarette breath, their alcohol hangovers, their blood pressure, or their cholesterol numbers. They don't want to lose ten years plus of their lives—missing on retirement, travelling, grandkids, volunteering for their church. They don't want to spend months on end recuperating from knee replacement or open heart surgery. They wish they liked fruits and vegetables a bit more, but carrots don't taste like pizza and, unfortunately, never will! However, they are willing to give five portions of fresh fruits and vegetables a day a really good try.

They do own a treadmill at home but, on most days, it simply collects dust. They go see their doctor to have their blood cholesterol tested and, maybe, they get a stress test. There are times they are seriously thinking about eating healthier and shaping up: increasing their physical activities and buying an activity tracker to count their daily steps. But when they see their peers—those who exercise daily, eat very carefully, and have little or no belly fat—they feel intimidated. Also, they may start taking seriously a worrisome family history—a heart attack of a younger sibling or colon cancer of a parent in his/her early sixties. They know they should do something about it. But the time never seems to be right for such a dramatic change. Too much stress at work and at home. And they are also afraid. Afraid of failure. Afraid of making a resolution, a commitment to themselves, a promise to others.

How can we help them?

For those in the middle of the road that want to change, a challenge lies ahead, but it is not as uphill as they may think. Yes, fear of change is real as is hesitation, procrastination, ice cream cravings, and fast food withdrawal. There will be setbacks. But if those who "crave" better health start the right way, many—if not most—will make it and they will love it! Here are some common patterns that prevent patients I see in my practice from improving their lifestyles:

- Some are not aware that their lifestyle is unhealthy. Almost every smoker knows that smoking is bad for his health, but a large number of individuals are not aware that they should be eating at least five portions of fruits and vegetables every day; that they should not be sitting for longer than six hours a day; that they should be doing at least 15,000 steps a day; and that they should sleep for a minimum of seven hours per night.

- Some are aware that their lifestyle is unhealthy but do not feel the need to improve it. They may feel they are either too young to be concerned about disease or too old to change. They smoke, they eat junk and processed food without fruits or vegetables, they have unhealthy snacks with added sugars, they drink sugary beverages, and they do not exercise. However, they like themselves they way they are and do not want to hear a word about changing.

- Some have thought about improving their lifestyle, but their resolution to change is still weak, overpowered by their habits and by feelings of intimidation caused by what they perceive as a very strict, limiting, and dull lifestyle.
- Some have thought about change and are willing to try. But they feel anxious and stressed over all the requirements of a healthy lifestyle. So, they try to find a stress-free period in their life to start their journey to a healthier self. When this doesn't happen (for personal, family, work, financial, or other reasons), their plans are abandoned.
- Some have tried in the past and failed (quit cigarettes and started again, lost weight, mostly through diet, and gained it back, started exercising but then stopped). Many are disappointed from their past failures and, although they would like to improve their lifestyle, they do not want to experience yet another failure.

My recommendations to such patients:

- For those who don't care to change, I remind them of what they are missing: an opportunity to get more "mileage" and better quality ride out of their ephemeral body. Health assets are at a maximum in our early twenties. With a healthy lifestyle and a bit of luck, we can maintain enough assets and live with minimum pain, suffering, disability, and need for surgeries into our seventies and beyond. Disrespect your health assets, and you may lose them (along with your life) by your forties or fifties.
- For those who have thought about improving their lifestyle but their commitment is not yet strong enough, I encourage them to do some soul searching, come up with the reasons why they want to change, and bring up any questions or concerns they may have.
- For those who are willing and determined to change, my advice is not to be intimidated by the strict requirements for a healthy diet or prolonged or strenuous physical activities. All they need is to start slow (remember, baby steps!), be very supportive of themselves, reward themselves for any improvement (no matter how small), not get discouraged when they have a setback, and remind themselves frequently why the want to change. They should allow themselves

a long horizon, measured in many months to a year or two for completing their lifestyle changes and not be intimidated by those who have already conquered a healthy lifestyle and have a great body figure. I ask them not to use the scale as the sole judge of success, as improvement in diet and exercise (or quitting smoking, for those who smoke) have a strong positive effect on their metabolism and artery health, even if they do not lose a single pound of weight.

- For those who have tried and failed, my recommendation is to be objective in analyzing the reasons behind the failure and not to get emotional. I remind them that setbacks are to be expected. Their responsibility is simply to get up and try again, armed with the experience of their previous efforts.

Start slow; it is baby steps that will get you where you want to go

Probably the most important piece of advice to those who are willing to improve their lifestyles is to start low and slow, without expecting perfection from the get go; you don't have to run a 10k on week one; nor do you need to eat six portions of fruits and vegetables by day 10. Guys, take your time, build your physical activities and nutritious habits, one small step at a time. Did I say small? No! One baby step at a time! And don't forget to show this positive energy, patting yourself in the back for every bit of achievement, no matter how small. You are not trying to beat a deadline or to prove anything to anyone. You only know why you do it. Avoid negative self-chatter. And leave plenty of room for those unavoidable setbacks and transgressions. No one is perfect, and any person who genuinely strives for the better deserves admiration and needs help, support, love, and understanding, not cold criticism, even if it comes from him or herself. Consider that for healthy lifestyle to work, it needs to:

- Be fun.
- Become a habit.
- Be your own free choice and at your own pace, not hastily or imposed by others
- Allow for occasional transgressions; when you fall, take a deep breath and stand up again as if nothing has happened.

Be persistent but patient

Be persistent but patient, and the reward will come. Consider that our natural state as humans, the state for which our bodies were originally built, is to stay physically active for several hours a day and eat fruits, vegetables, tubers, fish, and low-fat game. As we start our slow but steady return to this primal state of ours (we move more and eat better), there is a deep feeling of success and happiness. This wonderful and positive feeling is on top of the natural "high" that our endorphins create and will eventually make a healthy lifestyle easier to attain and maintain. This is one of the rewards of those who choose to follow a healthy lifestyle, not the momentary pleasure of gulping cookies and desserts, pizza, and burgers.

Don't let "trendy" dominate your life

Consider how much computers, cars, smartphones, chairs (yes, chairs), and washing machines have changed our everyday lives. And let's put processed food and bad carbs to the list. While all these tools and devices have allowed us to do unimaginable things at the stroke of a key and processed food has made meal preparation so much easier and faster, they have also led us astray from the primeval healthy lifestyle of our ancestors and into the limitless sitting, added sugars, and excessive salt abuse. Where can we find balance in a world that swirls at an ever increasing pace crushing everything that is not the "cutting-edge model" or the "latest fad"?

Find your inner voice

While external pressure is mounting, our inner voice can still tip the balance in our favor. Returning to our original path (remember the caveman) will make us feel content and proud. It is like what a mountaineer feels who, after struggling for days through a difficult and dangerous terrain, eventually, reaches the top of the mountain on a clear day with a breathtaking view of the lower land. That's also how we feel when we eventually lose 20 pounds (and keep them off), take our salad to work instead of falling for a cheeseburger, fattening desserts, and sugary beverages, complete 15,000 steps a day instead of 12 hours of sitting, and get ready for our first 5k running event instead of fantasizing about our next trip to the neighborhood pizzeria.

Say "No" to intimidation

You see people with perfect waistlines who exercise for hours daily, eat mostly fruits and vegetables, and very rarely consume red meat or desserts. You tell yourself: "I can never be like this!" And, in reality, you don't have to. In order to live healthy, you do not have to be perfect! There are no strict quotas and deadlines you must absolutely meet when you decide to live a healthier life. You may solicit the advice of your doctor, your dietician, and your personal trainer. These professionals are there to support you and guide you, not to issue penalties and ultimatums. And when you use the treadmill at the gym and feel exhausted after just ten minutes, while "Mr. Perfect" next to you has been running fast for over an hour, there is no reason to feel bad or intimidated. You are new to the healthy lifestyle; you are just starting while the other person may have been exercising for years and years. And most well-meaning healthy lifestylers will admire your efforts rather than judge you. And if you slip back a bit, activity- or diet-wise, there is no reason to feel ashamed, as long as you are willing to try again. **What is really bad is never giving healthy living a chance.**

Healthy living is anything but dull

Finally, for those who fear that practicing a healthy lifestyle means a "dull life without pleasures," think again. Take a look at people around you that are thin, athletic, and health-conscious. Do they look that unhappy and miserable to you? Allow yourself to experience the great feeling that your early small successes will offer you and the even greater feeling of, eventually, returning to a more pure and original way of life, a kind of return to your roots. Consider the daily struggles of our ancestors: they had to do so much physical work in order to find food and shelter. Their survival was not a given. Our modern life, in contrast, with most of the survival issues solved, with a safe home, a supermarket filled with all of God's goods, electricity and clean water, and warmth in the winter and cooling in the summer, offers convenience and security we take for granted. Where is the spirit and robustness of the survivors we used to be? By this, I do not mean we need to return to the stone age and adopt all Paleo and reject all modern. Rather, I express my skepticism over how much of what passes as a "given" way of life should we keep, how much we should reject, and how much we should change.

The good news is...

Here is more good news for those who aspire to improve their lifestyle: first, you are still alive and, hopefully, free of cancer, heart failure, or emphysema. Therefore, you are still in possession of a pretty good health capital. Second, as our bodies are built with tremendous reserves and a strong potential for self-healing, you are given a second chance, even after all those years that you didn't show your bodies the respect they deserved. Consider:

- We can survive and function well in spite of losing 50% of our lung or kidney function.
- Our heart can make ends meet with only two thirds of its power.
- Clogged heart or leg arteries can, over time, form thousands of tiny bypasses that allow blood to flow again through a previously 100 percent clogged artery.
- Our liver cells can regenerate.
- Our muscle can grow (there are individuals who became bodybuilders in their late sixties!).
- Our bone loss (after our forties) can be minimized through diet and exercise.
- Joint pain can be relieved with physical therapy and stretching exercises, without the need for surgery.

Your change helps all of us!

Beyond the benefits a healthier lifestyle brings to the individual, let's also look at the positive impact these middle-of-the-road people have on their families, their communities, and our country in general. These admirable people decide, after years of treating their bodies badly, to start taking better (not necessarily perfect) care of themselves.

We have an obligation to support and encourage them. These are the people who can return the tide in the obesity-diabetes-artery disease epidemic.

They represent a big hope, as they can get back on track and live a long, healthier life with less pain and suffering and fewer disabilities, medications, or procedures. This is a huge return on personal and societal investment. From the point of view of public health and health care spending, motivating those who don't practice a healthy lifestyle (and they are definitely the majority) to improve their health habits is where the money is. We should embrace the middle of the roaders with a sense of urgency and enthusiasm. These are opportunities and responsibilities for national and federal institutions, for local organizations, for schools and the workplace, and for other innovative, not yet existing modes of community activism.

Who's on your side?

The obesity-diabetes-artery disease epidemic cannot be fought just in hospitals and clinics by doctors and nurses. The same way, hospitals and clinics cannot be expected to motivate and support those in the middle of the road. These individuals are usually neither sick nor do they particularly enjoy any premature interaction with the health care establishment. They may actually avoid going to the doctor or they turn a deaf ear to the cold language of academicians and other scientists. While they seek change, they want it on their own terms and in their own territory. They are more likely to listen to the advice and encouragement of their friends and peers, their spouses and children, in real life encounters, or through social media and health blogs. When sound advice comes from friendlier and more down-to-earth sources, we tend to listen. The job of touting and promoting a healthy lifestyle in the community can only be accomplished by smart and innovative, community-driven, community-wide, and community-lead efforts.

The hurdles and the excuses: a summary

Health is such a complex issue that so many of us have serious misconceptions about it. And change is always a challenge, as old habits die hard. When faced with the challenge of changing their lifestyles, people often get emotional; they may completely withdraw from any further discussion or may come up with a myriad of excuses. And once emotions prevail, reasoning becomes futile.

Here is what I have heard from my patients over the years:

- Practicing healthy lifestyle is far too difficult for me; I am sure I am going to fail; I have tried it before, and it didn't work.
- Healthy lifestyle means hours of intense physical activity, and I do not have the stamina, the power, or the time to do it. I don't think I will ever be able to run half a marathon and, for this reason, healthy lifestyle is definitely not for me.
- I feel lazy; I don't have the motivation.
- My schedule is too busy; I don't have the time.
- I want to change but not now. I'll try maybe later, but definitely not now. I hope in a month or two conditions will be more favorable. Too much stress right now.
- I have a sedentary job; too much sitting. I have no muscles for the treadmill. Where should I start?
- I feel tired all the time.
- My joints hurt: my knees, my hips, my back. How am I supposed to exercise when everything hurts this bad?
- I like taking my time surfing on the net or watching TV when I am at home. You mean I should be walking on a treadmill while enjoying my favorite show?
- Exercise is boring and takes time away from fun activities.
- I don't want to exercise in front of others; I am ashamed of my body.
- I can't quit smoking. I have tried before and failed, more than once.
- I can't afford health club fees.
- I am afraid I might hurt myself with exercise.
- My family does not support my efforts.
- I have no time to cook at home or buy fresh ingredients.
- Fruits and vegetables are too expensive.
- Our cafeteria at work doesn't provide any tasty healthy choices.
- My family and I are allergic to healthy stuff.

If you really want to change to a healthy lifestyle, please be aware that:

- A small change is a huge achievement. Change your habits slowly, but be persistent and never give up.

- Adopting a healthy diet and the right amount of physical activity has its own learning curve; it cannot be learned overnight. Give yourself a few months to plan and implement a healthy lifestyle.
- Understand how stress forces us to resort to eating junk food that ends up destroying our health.
- You do not need to lose 40 pounds in 2 months; actually, losing weight is not a high priority, unless you are upwards of 300 pounds.
- You do not need to starve yourself.
- You do not need to run a half marathon every weekend.
- You do not need to become skinny like a supermodel or muscular like a bodybuilder.
- There is help; you must know someone among your friends, coworkers, or loved ones who has mastered a healthy lifestyle and has valuable tips for you.
- Don't be ashamed to exercise in front of others just because you are overweight or a beginner. You will draw much admiration for your resolve and efforts.
- Start slow: a few minutes of easy exercise along with a couple of fruits and a small salad a day is plenty for starters; build up gradually.
- Do not allow any negative self-talk, no matter how many setbacks you face. Maintain self-respect and confidence, rise up, and start all over again.
- You are there for the long-run. It may take months and years to see the results of your daily efforts. Don't weigh yourself daily, and do not allow the scale to be the only judge of your progress.

Changing in your twenties and thirties

If your lifestyle has been "so so," your spouse or friends have noticed a bulge in your belly (which is fat and not a pregnancy), and the number you see on the scale is less than thrilling, should you change? And how? You feel so young, though, and are so busy with life... Let me advise you that improving a less than healthy lifestyle early in life gives you the best possible chance to cruise through your forties and fifties, without the heart attacks or type 2 diabetes diagnoses of your peers, and spend your sixties and beyond without needing double knee replacement or a quadruple bypass surgery.

Losing weight is easier the younger you are, as:
- Your metabolic rate is still high.
- You have not yet lost significant amount of muscle or bone due to the aging process and your inactivity; your muscles, bones, and joints can support a pretty active lifestyle and even an intense exercise regimen, something you will not be able to do later in life.

Quitting smoking is also smart, as it is unlikely that you have a significant degree of emphysema by your late thirties. Also, within about three years from the time you quit smoking, your risk for artery disease goes down to the level of people who have never put a single cigarette in their mouth! Isn't this amazing?

In your twenties, your kidneys are so young that, even if you abuse salt, your blood pressure may still be normal. By your thirties, though, especially if you have any degree of belly fat, things change quite a bit. At that point, any extra salt you consume has a good chance to drive your blood pressure high, unless your genes are so wonderful that nothing will make you hypertensive before your sixties. If you do develop high blood pressure (above 140/90), you must remove salt from your diet, reduce animal fat, increase the amount of fruits and vegetables, and exercise on a daily basis (aim for close to 20,000 steps on your fitness tracker). Managing stress through meditation, praying, exercise, and social support also helps.

If these measures are not enough, you may need medications. With the obesity epidemic, even teenagers are not too young to develop high blood pressure and be in need of medications. Consider that your arteries will be damaged even at mild levels of blood pressure elevation (e.g., 150/95 mmHg) if those levels are sustained long enough. The concern about medication side effects should be balanced by an equal concern about high blood pressure "side effects" on your arteries, your heart, your kidneys, and your eyes. Consulting reputable websites (like World Health Organization, American Heart Association, American Society of Nephrology, NIH, Cleveland Clinic,and Mayo Clinic) will be an eye-opener for those with even mild blood pressure elevations. Yet, your best resource is your personal health care provider.

A mildly high LDL (the bad cholesterol) is not necessarily an indication for pills but should prompt you to decrease animal fat and sugars and increase the amount of fresh fruits, vegetables, whole grains, and foods that contain lots of fiber. Near daily exercise will also help. An LDL above 190 mg/dl is considered very high and is usually an indication for starting a statin (or other LDL-reducing therapies). Keep your A1c less than 5.7% and your fasting blood sugar less than 100 mg/dl if you can. If not, you have entered the world of prediabetes. This puts you to a whole different category. Forget free range of food choices and work closely with your healthcare provider. If not, you may be facing diabetes complications some 10 years down the road. See more about diabetes complications in chapters 1 and 2 .

Big threats to your health at this early stage in life are not only your abdominal obesity or your high blood pressure or cholesterol. You may also underestimate the risk these early deviations from metabolic and artery healthy pose later in life and have a false sense of security since "time is on your side." However, a fat belly can become type 2 diabetes, a high blood pressure can be the precursor of a stroke or kidney failure, and high cholesterol can lead to heart attacks or even sudden death over a decade or two.

Changing in your forties and fifties

If you have maintained a partially unhealthy lifestyle through your middle years, you must expect some degree of belly fat, insulin resistance, higher than normal blood pressure and triglycerides, fatty liver and fatty pancreas, and some knee pains due to arthritis. Your heart may be strong, but it is unlikely to relax normally (this heart stiffness is called "diastolic dysfunction" and is a common cause of shortness of breath when physically active). For smokers, some degree of emphysema is also common. All these changes, along with the passage of time, mean that cholesterol plaques are likely to be present in multiple locations in your arteries. When so many of my patients ask me the question: "Can these cholesterol plaques be flashed away?" the answer is "No." However, as long as those plaques remain stable, they will not threaten our lives, and it is much more likely to die with them than dying from them. This is why returning to as healthy a lifestyle as possible at any age will considerably boost your defence against heart attacks and stroke.

Having the early stages of metabolic, artery, and heart disease without the irreversible major catastrophes of heart attacks, stroke, and heart failure is exactly why there is still time to reap significant health benefits, should you start taking better care of your super high-tech body by:

- Eating healthy
- Quitting smoking
- Exercising, including opting for non-sitting arrangements at work for at least four hours a day
- Sleeping well
- Managing stress and keeping a healthy dose of optimism
- Avoiding alcohol or drug abuse
- Avoiding chronic use of NSAIDs or opioids
- Keeping a close relationship with your healthcare provider(s) and staying current on immunizations and screening tests.
- Knowing your "numbers" and monitoring your health

Changing in your sixties and beyond

If your lifestyle has been anything less than perfect, it is unlikely that you will reach your sixties without some degree of metabolic, artery, or heart disease and be entirely free of high blood pressure, prediabetes, abnormal cholesterol, or knee arthritis. If you have been a smoker, expect some degree of emphysema, as well. The benefits of changing to a healthy lifestyle at this point in life are still major, especially if you have not suffered a heart attack or stroke and have not developed heart failure or atrial fibrillation. See the previous paragraph for what lifestyle changes are the most important and most likely to help you increase both your life- and health-span.

By the time we reach our sixties or beyond, the effects of aging are obvious, even if our lifestyle has been close to perfect. Some degree of muscle and bone loss, knee or hip arthritis, high blood pressure, or prediabetes may be found even in those with the healthiest of lifestyles. What is then a major goal at this stage in life? Maintaining a good overall functional status, based on as good as possible functioning of your:

- Brain
- Heart and arteries
- Beta cells of your pancreas
- Muscles and bones
- Joints
- Kidneys
- Lungs
- Eyes

Exercise should be adapted to those forms of cardio, strengthening, stretching, and balancing that do not hurt your joints and do not cause you to become short of breath, dizzy, overly tired, or develop chest discomfort. Intense cardio exercises are particularly dangerous and should be avoided. Your sixties (or beyond) is not a time to run marathons, run hill sprints, or do 100-pound kettlebell swings. Walking, swimming, cycling, and water aerobics are much more appropriate forms of cardio exercises. Strengthening exercises, especially for your thigh muscles, are key to the ability to walk independently and safely, without falls (a major health hazard of the sixty-plus).

Keeping a rich and stimulating social life is extremely important. Don't stay home the entire day watching TV, or depression and strokes will soon follow. Especially for men, full retirement is a bad idea. Women always have something to do, but for men without hobbies, without a part time job, volunteering, or learning something new, a day has no structure and no meaning. Under these circumstances, the anticipated "paradise" of retirement may soon turn to hell.

Age-appropriate immunizations are also very important. For keeping up to date with immunizations, screenings (mammograms, pap smears, colonoscopies, prostate exams), and other preventive health issues, visiting your health care provider only once a year may not be enough. Since your health care visits may be more frequent, choose your providers wisely. Find the ones you can relate well with, that understand you and give you time to express your concerns and ask key questions. However, don't expect your doctor to answer 10 questions in one visit, given current healthcare constraints of ever-decreasing reimbursement.

For those who are happy as middle of the roaders

Suppose you smoke or drink more than a couple of beers a day and are determined that you are not going to stop. However, you are willing to walk for half an hour three times a week and give a chance to a couple of fruits and a small salad a day (without giving up your steak, burger, ice cream, or donut). If you are one of those middle of the roaders that are just happy the way they are, be aware that every bit of additional physical activity, every additional fruit or salad, every one less donut, cookie, or salted bread stick and butter at the restaurant will give you a better shot at a longer and healthier life. If you love fast food, you will be better off having fast food every other day instead of every day. Walking a mere 10 minutes per day is better than never exercising. If you cannot do without your six pack of beer, binging once a week is better than drinking 12 beers every day. However, smoking and artery/heart disease is an unusual exception: smoking only two cigarettes gives you almost the same risk for heart attacks as smoking two packs of cigarettes a day. Of course, the risk of emphysema, lung, throat, and bladder cancer is higher the more cigarettes you smoke, but it is worthwhile noticing that the risk of heart attacks is not brought down till we completely quit.

For anyone who is interested in some, no matter how small, improvement towards a healthier lifestyle, here are some additional tips:
- Long-lasting change is more likely when you are self-motivated and think positively.
- Goals are easier to reach if they're specific: "I'll walk 10 minutes today" rather than "I'll start exercising."
- Having too many goals is counterproductive; you cannot afford to devote to each one of those the willpower you can devote to just one.
- It's not enough to have a goal; you also need practical and realistic ways to reach it.

Setting easy and realistic goals is a smart strategy:
- It is easier to decide to start exercising when you know you will not be "torturing" yourself for hours; 5 or 10 minutes of light exercise is not going to kill you!

- You are far more likely to succeed when your early goals are easy. Setting the bar too high on day 1 of your "new and healthier life" may lead to injuries, failures, and disappointments, and you may quit altogether.
- You will get tremendous encouragement by your early success and may decide to go for more. You may exercise for just 10 minutes a day every other day for the first two to three weeks and build up gradually. Within two to six weeks, your muscles, heart, and lungs will get adjusted and help you get to the next level as if it were a breeze!

Healthy Tuesday

If eating healthy and exercising every day conjures images from Dante's "Inferno," it may be more comforting to decide to "torture" yourself just one day a week. Think it over during the weekend and get prepared mentally. Budget some time; clear your schedule; turn your cell phone off. And start on a Tuesday. Tuesday sounds like a good choice; there is too much stress on Mondays, and Wednesday is so far removed from your weekend health resolution, you might forget it altogether. And go gentle. A few minutes of an easy workout, a healthy breakfast, five portions of fresh fruits and vegetables, and a dinner prepared by you from real food ingredients. That's it! Repeat it over a few weeks, and see whether you can add a second day, a "healthy Thursday," for example. Before you know it, YOU ARE practicing a healthy lifestyle—maybe part time and light so far, but you are a success. And, please, do not jump on the scale. This is far too early to expect any weight loss. Your goal is to take the mystery and the fear of the unknown out of the healthy lifestyle and start practicing it easily, naturally, and make it fun. Within a few months, your body will be asking for more of the "good stuff," and you will be practicing a healthy lifestyle consistently before you know it!

Not exercising because of having no money for a home treadmill or a gym membership is just an excuse. Here are some alternatives that come at no additional cost, provided that you own or rent a home:
- Marching in place
- Using resistance bands

- Pushups or squats
- Extending your arms
- Simple stretching
- Yoga exercises, available for free on the internet

Don't be impatient

Once you decide to change your lifestyle for the healthier, practice it daily without looking at the scale or measuring your waist circumference or blood pressure three times a day. The art of living healthy day in and day out takes practice and a long time to be perfected. Even after it is mastered, healthy lifestyle takes some time to increase your stamina and improve the function of your heart, lungs, muscles, and liver so that, eventually, both your metabolism and your cardiovascular function is improved. So, be patient. It takes time. Don't expect instant gratification. Stay focused, persevere, reward yourself for your early successes, no matter how small, and rest assured that the journey will be worthwhile.

Don't let the scale be the only judge

Losing weight, while important if you have belly fat, prediabetes, high blood pressure, or diabetes, cannot be the only parameter that tells success from failure as you try to live healthier. For one, not smoking, eating healthy, and exercising adequately every day are more important in improving your metabolism and artery health compared to simply losing weight. Second, losing weight can be very difficult to accomplish or may take months of healthy lifestyle before you shed (and keep off) that dreaded first pound.

Maintaining a healthy weight after some early weight loss can also prove a greater challenge than losing the weight in the first place. Please consider that weight loss, while desirable, is not the ultimate criterion of success as we try to improve our lifestyle. The ultimate proof of success of any wellness or prevention measure is living longer without pain, suffering, and disability. And you can achieve this goal by living healthy every day, even if you don't lose a single pound.

And if you never manage to achieve a 100 percent healthy lifestyle, don't give up; practicing a healthy lifestyle 10 percent of the time is much better than not practicing it at all, and 20 percent is definitely better than 10 percent. Inviting healthy lifestyle, even part time, into your life allows you to become familiar with it and not dread it, opening the door for more healthy stuff in the future.

Chapter 5 Questions

1. For which of the following individuals who have been smoking since their late teens is too late to quit smoking?
   - A 40-year-old woman with chronic bronchitis
   - A 55-year-old man with emphysema
   - An apparently healthy 30-year-old woman
   - A 70-year-old woman with bladder cancer
   - A 65-year-old man who was just diagnosed with lung cancer
   - None of the above

2. A 40-year-old man has been eating fast food all his life. He never eats fruits. He occasionally eats a salad. You advise him to gradually start eating more fruits and vegetables so that he eventually eats at least five portions of fruits and vegetables a day. He tells you that it is impossible to do this during the workdays due to his stress but he can try it over the weekend. Assuming he succeeds, is this a meaningful improvement of his lifestyle?

3. You advise a 60-year-old obese woman who has never exercised in her life (but is willing to give it a try) to start an exercise program. She tells you that she has knee arthritis and cannot walk without a cane. She cannot afford a gym membership, so swimming or water aerobics are out of the way. Should she give up on exercise?

4. A 52-year-old man is discharged from the hospital after a quadruple bypass surgery. He is obese (weight circumference 48 inches), but he has never smoked. He was diagnosed with type 2 diabetes 10 years ago. His blood pressure is 140/80 mmHg on three blood pressure pills. He works two jobs, both sedentary. He has never exercised, but he is willing to try, although time allotted for leisure is about 10–20 minutes a day, due to his busy work schedule. He has less than five hours to sleep at night. He has three young kids. He wants to live to see them grow up, and he is willing to do anything possible to improve his health. What is the single most effective

change in his lifestyle than can help his health improve in the long run?

5. You are a 35-year-old woman. Your BMI is 32, and your waist circumference is 38 inches, so you are obese. Your A1c is 6%, so you are prediabetic (your dad had diabetes). Your blood pressure is 140/90 mmHg. Your job involves sitting in front of a computer 10 hours a day. Commuting to and from work takes one hour (sitting). You have no time to exercise, and you eat heavily processed, unhealthy meals. You decide to start living healthy, buy a standing desk for work, prepare meals from fresh ingredients, move more at work, and add some exercise, too. Your fitbit registers 15,000 steps a day. You lift moderate weights every other day. Six months later, your A1c is 5.5% and your blood pressure is 130/82. Your waist circumference is 36 inches but your weight has remained the same. You are disappointed that, after so much hard work, you haven't lost a single pound. You feel that all your efforts were wasted as the scale shows zero weight loss. Are you right to feel this way?

6. You are in your early sixties, abdobese, sedentary, and a smoker. Your family doctor, after two years' attempts, persuades you to quit smoking, eat healthy, and start exercising. You lose significant weight on the way. Beyond reducing your risk for developing diabetes, heart attacks, leg gangrene, and stroke, your risk for developing which of the following diseases also goes down?
    *   Cancer
    *   Alzheimer's
    *   Emphysema
    *   Knee arthritis
    *   All of the above

Chapter 6

WHAT IS A HEALTHY LIFESTYLE?

"Health is not simply the absence of sickness."
—Hannah Green

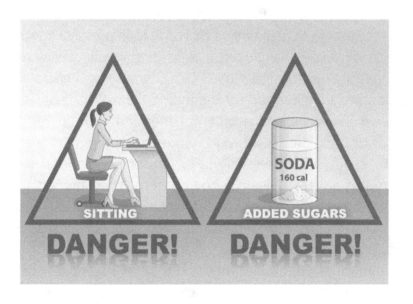

The obesity-diabetes-artery disease epidemic kills people, ravages lives and families, weakens the labor force, costs almost a trillion dollars every year, and undermines our society. Yet the epidemic is largely preventable by adopting a healthier lifestyle. How, then, do we allow such a simple solution (that is, practicing a healthy lifestyle consistently) to stand in the way of solving such major a problem of our times as the obesity-diabetes-artery disease epidemic is? And if we practice this healthy lifestyle, what other diseases, beyond those involved in the obesity-diabetes-artery disease epidemic, can we expect to also prevent? Finally, what exactly is a healthy lifestyle? These are the questions that Chapter 6 will attempt to answer.

A key cause of the obesity epidemic (and the main reason we have, so far, been unsuccessful in defeating it) is that, due to impressive advancements in technology, we have developed a lifestyle that was not in store for us and our bodies. Our ancestors of 100,000 years ago had to work hard for their food and shelter and for defending themselves against invaders and wild animals. While the cavemen's genes and their offsprings looked very similar to ours, they were much leaner and more muscular than we are today. Activity-wise, they walked or ran for two to four hours every day, seven days a week. They climbed on trees. They jumped. They lifted stones. They ate a diverse diet consisting of wild game, free range grass-fed meat, wild caught fish, and plants, food that was available but not abundant, and was devoid of salt or added sugars. They craved sugars and fats as much as we do, but they had to work had to get them. And if hunting went well and food was available for a couple of days, they would take that time off; when there was no necessity or incentive to do physical work, they would stay home and rest, just like we do.

Our technological advancements and innovations changed our daily lives so fast that there was no time for our bodies to adapt. Therefore, today:

- We live in suburbia and use automobiles to go to our workplace, the grocery store, and wherever we spend our leisure time.
- Kids play games on their smartphones instead of playing outside.
- At the workplace, the successful modern employee, sitting for 10–12 hours a day in front of a computer, can be 100 percent productive and 100 percent sedentary.

- At home we spend several hours sitting while watching screen-based (TV, computer, tablet, smartphone) entertainment or continue working.
- Frequent deadlines and demands for ever higher productivity make us feel stressed. To escape, we indulge in tasty foods and snacks, especially sugary foods and drinks, which cause insulin spikes and make us hungry within less than two hours. In other words, we are in an almost continuous state of munching unhealthy foods.
- While our craving for sugars and animal fats has not changed since the time of the caveman, we can now find these calorie-dense, fiber-deprived delicacies at affordable prices in almost all stores (not only in supermarket aisles) after a short ride in the car.
- The meat we now eat comes frequently from corn-fed beef, cage-raised chicken, and farm-raised fish and has much more fat than the meat consumed by our ancestors.
- We consider our lifestyle "physically active" if we walk 30 minutes a day, five days a week. Nearly 50 percent of us are meeting even this minimum physical activity level.

Switching to a healthier lifestyle that requires much more body movement and healthier but less tasty foods is simple but at the same time so difficult, as it goes against our own "software":

- If there is no need to move my body and get out of my comfortable chair, why should I do it? The caveman would have done exactly the same!
- And if food is easily available and tasty, why should I not eat it? The caveman would have done exactly the same!

And in this, we are right: presented with the same set of social conditions at home, the workplace, and the grocery store, the caveman would have behaved exactly like us. And he would have become obese and diabetic and most likely would have died of heart disease or cancer, the same way we do.

Our instincts push us to avoid the "discomfort" of physical activity and choose the comfort of sitting when we do not have to put hard physical labor in order to find food and shelter or create and sustain a family. No wonder that, thanks to our own success in technological innovations that make everyday life "easier," we live in the time of obesity, type 2 diabetes, and artery disease.

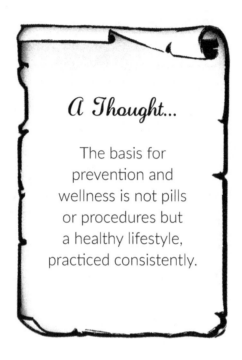

A Thought...

The basis for
prevention and
wellness is not pills
or procedures but
a healthy lifestyle,
practiced consistently.

This chapter, while focusing on the prevention of the obesity-diabetes-artery disease epidemic, also includes basic principles of a healthy lifestyle that help in the prevention of many top killer diseases in our country.

Here is a list of the **top 10 causes of death**, the worst killer diseases for adults in the US:

1. **Heart and Artery Disease**
2. **Cancer**
3. Unintentional injuries (including the rising tide of **opioid overdose**)
4. **Chronic lung disease**
5. **Stroke**
6. **Alzheimer's disease**
7. **Diabetes**
8. **Pneumonia** and influenza
9. **Kidney disease**
10. Suicide

The same principles of healthy lifestyle that help prevent obesity, diabetes, and heart and artery disease can also be applied to the prevention of almost 50 percent of cancers, most chronic lung disease (emphysema, chronic bronchitis, chronic asthma), stroke, many cases of Alzheimer's and pneumonia, and most cases of chronic kidney disease. The case of **Alzheimer's,** a signature disease of the 20th and 21st century and another global epidemic and costly chronic disease whose rate is still rising, is particularly interesting; out of all the **risk factors for Alzheimer's, there is only one that is not included in the prevention of obesity, diabetes, and artery disease,** namely **head trauma at any point in life,** through sports injuries or bike/ motor vehicle accidents.

What is included in this chapter is a more thorough approach to what a healthy lifestyle is and covers:

- Not smoking
- Healthy diet
- Prolonged moderate-intensity physical activity throughout the day
- Adequate and high-quality sleep
- Preservation of the day-night cycle
- Avoiding unnatural stress
- Limiting work to 55 hours per week
- Avoiding chronic use of NSAIDs and opioids
- Avoiding alcohol abuse
- Avoiding drug use
- Avoiding weight gain
- Obtaining age- and disease-appropriate immunizations
- Choosing the right vitamins
- Embracing helpful screening procedures
- Having a not-giving-up attitude
- Having a rich social life
- Living for a reason

Healthy lifestyle adds years to your life and happiness to your years. It helps you avoid unnecessary pain, suffering, and disability; it minimizes your need of medications and procedures; it cuts your medical bills and insurance premiums; and makes our society healthier and more robust. But for a healthy lifestyle to work, it needs to become a habit and fun. You should be able to, naturally and without having to think or push yourself, make the right food choices, stay active at the workplace and at home, regularly enjoy a full night's sleep, avoid tobacco and alcohol abuse, and find a balance between work, family, and personal time.

In this chapter, we will clarify what a healthy lifestyle really is by spelling out its key elements. And while the focus is on avoidance of obesity, diabetes, and artery disease, some other elements, like immunizations and screening tests, are also mentioned. However, this chapter makes no claim of covering every aspect of healthy living.

Not smoking

Tobacco smoking releases about 7,000 chemicals, not just nicotine and tar. Some of these chemicals are radioactive gases (no wonder smoking causes cancer of the lungs, neck, throat, mouth, esophagus, stomach, liver, pancreas, colon, rectum, cervix, and bladder). Smoking also causes lung disease (emphysema and chronic bronchitis) and is a key trigger of asthma. Smoking is one of the most powerful ways to destroy one's arteries through the development of cholesterol plaque disease. In addition, smoking products raise the blood pressure, speed up the heart rate, and make the arteries more likely to go into spasm and artery clots more likely to happen.

According to the National Cancer Institute, there is no safe level of tobacco use. People who use any type of tobacco products should quit. People who quit smoking, regardless of their age, gain substantially in life expectancy compared with those who continue to smoke. Even quitting smoking at the time of a cancer diagnosis reduces the risk of death.

Chewing tobacco and smokeless tobacco can cause cancer of the esophagus, mouth, throat, cheek, gums, lips, tongue, and pancreas. It also results in bad smell, cavities, tooth decay, and gum disease.

Healthy diet

Is your diet an asset for your health or a liability?

Consider that there are only three types of food (besides water) that are nutritious and necessary for our survival:

- Fruits, vegetables, and whole grains (as they provide fiber, vitamins, and energy)
- Lean protein (skinless poultry, low-fat dairy, legumes, soy, hemp)
- Good fats (olive and canola oils, unsalted nuts, salmon, sardines, flaxseed, avocado, and dark chocolate)

We need to consume large quantities of the good carbs (diabetics should avoid some high-sugar fruits like watermelon, grapes, and figs), moderate quantities (about 40–70 gm a day) of lean protein, and small quantities of good fats (as they are calorie dense—9 calories per gram). If you are using olive oil, vinegar, and lemon on your salad, you are on the right path. If you are using store-bought salad dressings, you are on your own!

Healthy diet helps us meet the energy needs of our body and provides additional protection against diabetes, artery disease, and cancer through antioxidants and fiber. In spite of the fact that calories are calories, from the point of view of providing energy, not all calories are created equal regarding protection against diabetes, artery disease, and cancer.

Added sugars and fast food define a morbid but, unfortunately, deeply rooted diet culture. Fast foods provide energy without providing enough antioxidants or fiber; instead, they put into our bodies dangerous chemicals like saturated and trans fats and bad carbs ("high glycemic index" carbs). These bad carbs stress out our pancreas' beta cells as they demand a quick insulin spike to match the sugar spike in the bloodstream. This is not the case with good carbs, like fruits, veggies, and whole grains, which allow sugar absorption to take place only gradually, are gentle to the pancreas, and help us avoid insulin spikes. Insulin spikes are not only bad because of stressing our pancreas. As refined sugars are digested quickly, they cause a mild hypoglycemia (lowering of blood sugar) about two hours after they are ingested. This leads to blood sugar swings and cravings, making it more difficult to control our overall calorie intake. Bad carbs put us in a vicious cycle: our hunger is satisfied by bad carbs ("comfort food!"), causing more hunger two hours later to be, again, satisfied by more bad carbs, and so on, till our belly becomes a huge glob of fat.

These are the foods and substances our body does not need:

Bad Carbs:
- White bread, white pasta, and white rice
- Cookies, donuts, desserts, and candies
- Sugary beverages
- Cereals with lots of added sugars
- "Low-fat" foods with lots of added sugars, as they tend to be high in carbs. Look for "sugars" when you buy "low-fat" yogurt. Low-fat foods may even contain trans-fats, also labeled as "hydrogenated fats" or "shortening."
- We can survive without ever eating white bread, white pasta, white rice, or cookies. Just keep this in mind!

Bad Fats:
- Skin of poultry
- French fries
- Fast food
- Potato chips
- Milk chocolate
- Whole fat milk
- Fatty cheese like brie
- Ice cream
- Butter or lard
- Beef, pork, or lamb more than twice a week
- Coconut oil
- Margarine sticks

Avoid trans fats, the most dangerous fat that exists

Trans fats are created artificially by adding hydrogen to liquid vegetable oils to make them solid. In this way, trans fats are easier to use, inexpensive to produce, and last for a long time. They also make foods tastier and give them a nice, crunchy texture. However, trans fats have a detrimental effect on our blood cholesterol, as they raise our bad (LDL) cholesterol and lower our good (HDL) cholesterol. These trans fat effects significantly increase our risk of developing type 2 diabetes and artery disease.

Do you know that manufacturers are allowed to list as "0 grams" any quantity that is less than 0.5 grams per serving? They are also allowed to define as "serving size" the smallest quantity that contains 0 trans fats and as few as possible calories, sodium-salt, and saturated fats. The Cleveland Clinic Guide to trans fats warns that the following foods are likely to include significant amounts of these dangerous fats, even if their food label mentions "0 grams of trans fat" (cakes, pies, and cookies).

- Biscuits
- Breakfast sandwiches
- Some margarine sticks or tubs
- Crackers
- Some microwave popcorn
- Cream-filled candies
- Donuts
- Fried fast foods
- Frozen pizza

"Comfort" food

Say "comfort food," and images of apple pie, chocolate chip cookies, ice cream, M&Ms, potato chips, or pizza may come to mind. Scientific research has shown what many of us already know from personal experience: when under stress, we are more vulnerable and more likely to make unhealthy food choices. Foods that contain sugar, fats, and lots of calories are more likely to be used as comfort food, as compared to carrots, celery, or tomatoes. However, at the end of the day (or night) of binging on unhealthy but "comfort" food, it is not surprising that so many of us feel guilt instead of comfort!

Coffee

Coffee is a necessity for so many of us. And there is good scientific evidence that, up to a limit, coffee is actually good for our health. It contains antioxidants that prevent cell damage, and a 2012 study in *New England*

Journal of Medicine found that consumption of coffee was associated with lower risk of death from heart disease, diabetes, stroke, respiratory disease, infections, and even accidents and injuries. There is some (although debatable) scientific evidence that drinking more than four cups of regular caffeinated coffee daily may be a health risk, associated with higher mortality, especially for individuals younger than 55 years of age.

There are some individuals whose blood pressure may increase after drinking coffee; these individuals should limit their consumption. Recommendations about limited use of coffee include pregnant women (no more than two cups of coffee per day) and adolescents (no more than one cup daily).

It is important to add that smokers consume higher amounts of coffee than non-smokers. If you consider the negative health effects of smoking along the positive effects of coffee, smoking hazards unfortunately win. So, if you are a smoker who believes that you cannot enjoy a cup of coffee without lighting up a cigarette, you may be better off giving up coffee if this makes you more likely to smoke less or quit altogether.

Prolonged, moderate-intensity physical activity throughout the day

Single line exercise recommendation: "Perpetual, non-injurious movement with periods of rest in between (sitting or lying down)"

Man was made for Paleo fitness activities like:
- Six to nine miles a day on uneven terrain, every day
- Lifting and throwing stones
- Climbing on trees
- Repairing frequent injuries (not a fitness activity by itself but burning a whole lot of calories)

This translates to our present-day culture as:
- Two to four hours of walking-like cardio
- 15+ minutes of strengthening (weights or rubber bands, for example)

- 15+ minutes of stretching and balancing exercises (simple stretching, yoga, or tai-chi)

Which comes up to a total of 2.5 to 4.5 hours a day. So, it appears that the difference between what we think is adequate physical activity and what truly IS the recommended physical activity is huge! By recommending at least of 30 minutes of walking, five days a week, physician organizations might have inadvertently lowered the bar way too much!

It is important to recognize that while cardio ("aerobic" exercise) is the basis of physical activities, it is definitely not enough. Strengthening exercises are a must, as physical inactivity and aging result in loss of muscle. Our dwindling muscle mass, in turn, results in a slower metabolism and makes it easier to gain weight. Not only this, but later in life, no muscle means no independence; so many of us in our sixties and beyond end up having thighs that consist of 80 percent fat, with just a toothpick of muscle and bone in the middle. It's no surprise that people with few muscles complain that their legs feel "so heavy"! Fat cannot lift our bodyweight; only muscle can! There is a reason the Creator made our bodies consisting of 40–50 percent muscle. That muscle is there to be used. On any opportunity we can get! Daily!

On top of cardio and strengthening exercises, we also need stretching and balancing exercises (yoga, tai-chi, simple stretching). These exercises are necessary in order to keep our joints flexible and healthy and to prevent falls later in life. Consider that if our joints (knees, hips, back, shoulders) hurt, we cannot use our muscles; we cannot walk or exercise, but we can still eat and gain inordinate amounts of weight. Additionally, if our joints hurt, we are likely to take painkillers. Some of them (NSAIDs like ibuprofen or naproxen) are dangerous when taken daily, as they can cause our kidneys and hearts to fail, our blood pressure and potassium to soar, our ankles to swell, and our stomachs to hurt or even bleed. Also, they will make you retain a few pounds of unnecessary fluid. Other medications (opioids, like methadone and oxycontin) can make us sleepy the whole day, reduce our level of activities, and cause falls or disturbed sleep patterns and are addictive. Sleep apnea is dangerous, as not only does it result in unrefreshing sleep, but it also contributes to heart attacks, high blood pressure, and heart failure. When considering an over-the-counter painkiller, acetaminophen (the ingredient in Tylenol) is a safer choice when used as directed (no more than 2 grams a day for most of the time and never more than 4 gm in any 24 hour period, as it can cause liver failure), but it is frequently not strong enough to quell our arthritis pains.

While physical activity is vital for our health, we should not overdo it. Running half a marathon every weekend or exercising for more than four or five hours a day can destroy your joints; then you are stuck with arthritis for the rest of your life. Excessive exercise can also cause cessation of the normal menstrual cycle in young women. While non-sitting arrangements at work are very much desirable, standing for more than four hours a day can cause back pain and varicose veins in your legs. Everything in moderation!

Adequate and high-quality sleep

We need to sleep the same way we need to eat and drink. Most adults need seven to nine hours of sleep every night. If you sleep only four to five hours a day because you "cannot afford" longer sleeping hours, be aware that you are depriving your body of one of its most essential health ingredients. During sleep, the brain rests, gets rid of waste, and repairs wear and tear. In children and adolescents, sleep is essential for growth and development. Sleep deprivation is dangerous to your mental and physical health and can dramatically lower your quality (and quantity) of life. While sleepiness, yawning, and irritability are some of the most obvious effects of sleep deprivation, its real price is much higher.

Here are some serious consequences of depriving your body of adequate and high-quality uninterrupted sleep:
- Lower ability to fight infections and chronic illness
- Increased risk for falls due to worsening balance and coordination
- Reduced ability to concentrate and learn; reduced creativity
- Short temper, irritability, and mood swings
- Increased risk for potentially lethal accidents

Inadequate, frequently interrupted or low-quality sleep Increases the risk for developing a host of chronic illnesses like:

- Obesity
- Metabolic syndrome
- High blood pressure
- Type 2 diabetes
- Atrial fibrillation
- Stroke
- Depression

So, if, for any reason (working long hours, playing games incessantly or staying up all night watching TV out of boredom), you stint on sleep, you risk serious damage to your physical and mental health. In particular, sleep deprivation due to long working hours is both serious and difficult to recognize, as hard work is seen in our culture as a positive trait. We believe that all good things come at a price and are eager to accept shorter sleep for the projected benefits of our hard work. So, there is a real risk to our health when we believe that the positive effects of hard work outweigh the negative effects of sleep deprivation. Considering how dangerous—even lethal—sleep deprivation can be, we need to have a serious discussion with ourselves about the reasons that make us devote long hours to work. Is it worth it?

Work and play during the day; sleep during the night

A close "relative" to sleep deprivation is working the night shift. Shift work can result in the so called "shift work disorder," caused by night shifts, ro-tating shifts, or even a very early (before 6:00 a.m.) morning shift. It can cause chronic sleep deprivation, in which a person never catches up on needed sleep and carries a significant "sleep debt." This kind of chronic loss of sleep has serious implications for health, productivity, and safety. The day and night rhythm in living organisms was deemed so important that the **2017 Nobel prize** for Physiology or Medicine was awarded to three US scientists for their discoveries of molecular mechanisms controlling the **circadian rhythm.**

Excessive sleepiness and "microsleeps"

According to the National Sleep Foundation, many shift workers struggle with not only headaches, irritability, lack of energy, and difficulty concentrating, but also with excessive sleepiness during the hours in which they're supposed to be at work, with family, or during leisure activities. The symptom of excessive sleepiness means that you feel as though you're fighting sleep during work or social time. This excessive sleepiness goes beyond the natural "dip" in alertness that many of us may feel at certain points in the day and becomes a near-constant symptom that interferes with our ability to work, drive, or socialize. There is a big price to pay when we go against the body's natural cycle of "be active during the day, but sleep at night."

"Microsleep" is a brief sleep that happens to people who are sleep-deprived. Although it lasts for only a few seconds, it can be very dangerous if it happens in front of an assembly line or while driving or operating machinery. What are the consequences of shift work sleep disorder?
- Increased accidents
- Increased work-related errors
- Increased sick leave
- Increased irritability or mood problems

When left untreated, shift work disorder can not only cause decreased productivity and interpersonal problems, but it can also contribute to high blood pressure and heart disease, digestive problems, and depression.

Sleep deprivation

"So many people are sleep-deprived," says Carol Ash, DO, medical director of Sleep for Life, a sleep disorders treatment program in Hillsborough, NJ. "We're living in a time of unprecedented sleep debt." It doesn't help that we've evolved into a 24/7 society. Two hundred years ago, people used to go to bed when the sun went down. Now, technology has allowed us to turn night into day. Human physiology can't keep up with that. "People sacrifice sleep to get more and more done," Dr. Ash continues.

Dr. James Walsh, MD, director of the St. John's Mercy Sleep Medicine and Research Center in St. Louis comments: "Our round-the-clock lifestyles come at a big cost. The ability to think, concentrate, remember and problem-solve deteriorates as we become sleep-deprived."

Sleep strategies

"There are a lot of things that interfere with sleep," says Dr. Paul Selecky, MD, medical director of the Hoag Sleep Disorders Center in Newport Beach, CA, on healthcommunities.com. "But most are of our own doing." Try these good-sleep measures to turn the tide:

- Establish a relaxing bedtime routine, such as taking a warm bath.
- Make your bedroom as quiet, dark, and comfortable as possible. Consider blackout curtains, earplugs, a sleep mask, fans, or white-noise machines.
- Eliminate caffeine, alcohol, and nicotine, particularly late in the day.
- Exercise, but not close to bedtime (do not exercise after 9:00 p.m., unless you perform simple stretching or yoga).
- Quell your worries before you try to fall asleep. To clear your mind well before you head to bed, devote a half hour to worrying.
- Don't try to sleep unless you are tired. In bed, read a book or listen to music until you feel drowsy.
- If you don't doze off in 20 minutes, get out of bed and do something relaxing until you're sleepy.
- Get up at the same time each morning, even on weekends and holidays.
- Use your bedroom only for sleep and intimacy.

Avoiding unnatural stress

The usual stress of the caveman was running for his life, hunting for food, finding shelter, or facing a natural disaster; it was intense and life-threatening but brief. And the caveman's response to this stress was not only beneficial, it was lifesaving. Modern man does not often face this intense but short lived stress of running for his life. Rather, it is financial worries, deadlines, demanding and unreasonable bosses, chronic work stress, stifling traffic, difficult situations at home. All these make us feel nervous, hopeless, or depressed. This chronic, lingering, sustained type of stress is unnatural, and it can truly affect both our physical and psychological health.

Randolph Nesse, MD and Elizabeth Young, MD summarize the social and mental threats of modern man in the following statement: "Most stresses in modern life arise not from physical dangers or deficiencies, but from our tendency to commit ourselves to personal goals that are too many and too high. When our efforts to accomplish these goals are thwarted or when we cannot pursue all the goals at once and must give something up, the stress reaction is expressed. In short, much stress arises, ultimately, not from a mismatch between our abilities and the environment's demand, but from a mismatch between what we desire and what we can have." Research shows that social conditions—the jobs we do, the money we are paid, the schools we attend, the neighborhoods we live in—are as important to our health as our genes, our behaviors, and even our medical care. It is well established that life stress can significantly contribute to ill health among vulnerable individuals.

Limit work to no more than 55 hours per week

There is scientific evidence that working too long is dangerous for our health. While our society values hard work, our bodies deliver a different verdict. A study led by scientists at the University College in London and published in *Lancet* in 2015 found that those who work more than 55 hours per week have a 33% increased risk of stroke and 13% increased risk of heart artery disease, as compared with those who limit their working hours to no more than 40 per week. Other studies have found that long working hours are associated with increased risk of developing type 2 diabetes, depression, heart attacks, sleep disorders, and alcohol abuse. Science raises a red flag and adds the habit to work for longer than 55 hours per week to the list of unhealthy behaviors like smoking and skimping on sleep.

In spite of the long-entrenched positive attitudes towards long working hours, healthy lifestyle suggests otherwise. We are responsible adults and we should be making informed decisions, fully aware of the short- and long-run consequences.

Avoid chronic use of NSAIDs and opioids

Near-daily use of these drugs for months or years on end can be very dangerous to your health. NSAIDs are popular painkillers and anti-inflammatory medications available over the counter in the US. Generics include ibuprofen, naproxen, piroxicam, diclofenac, celecoxib, indomethacin, and meloxicam. Brand names include Motrin and Advil (ibuprofen), Aleve, Anaprox, Naprosyn (naproxen), Feldene (piroxicam), Voltaren (diclofenac), Celebrex (celecoxib), Indocin (indomethacin), and Mobic (meloxicam).

While NSAIDs are very effective in controlling arthritis and other types of pain, their frequent (near-daily) use can cause heart attacks, heart failure, kidney failure, high blood pressure, high potassium, stomach ulcers, and gastrointestinal bleeding. Patients with kidney disease or health conditions predisposing to kidney disease (like diabetes and high blood pressure) should generally avoid these medications altogether. Aspirin is also an anti-inflammatory medication, but, except for stomach ulcers and gastrointestinal bleeding, not only does it not cause heart attacks, but it is used in the prevention of both heart attacks and stroke. If ever, NSAIDs should be taken with a full stomach and while the patient is well hydrated and for the shortest period possible.

Popular opioid analgesic medications include generics like codeine, fentanyl (brand name: Duragesic), hydrocodone (available in combination with acetaminophen as Vicodin, Norco, and Lortab), morphine (MS Contin), oxycodone (OxyContin and, in combination with acetaminophen as Percocet), methadone, and meperidine (Demerol). These medications are effective against several forms of moderate and severe pain and are more potent than acetaminophen (Tylenol). They are acceptable as short-course treatment of acute pain and pain in terminally ill (for example, advanced, metastatic cancer) patients. When used for other indications and taken near-daily for longer than a week, they can cause addiction. Beyond sedation and constipation, they can also cause low-quality, disrupted sleep ("central sleep apnea"), which can lead to high blood pressure and heart attacks.

According to the Substance Abuse and Mental Health Services Administration (SAMHSA), opiate use disorder involves:

- Strong desire to use opioids
- Inability to control or reduce use
- Trouble meeting social or work obligations
- Having legal problems due to drug use
- Spending large amounts of time to obtain opiates
- Development of tolerance
- Having withdrawal symptoms after stopping or reducing use

Avoid alcohol abuse

If you use alcohol, do so in moderation and avoid alcohol abuse. There is good scientific evidence that small-to-moderate amounts of regular alcohol intake are good for our health. However, alcohol in more than moderate amounts becomes a poison.

The recommended limits of alcohol intake are:

- No more than two drinks per 24 hours for men up to the age of 65
- No more than one drink per 24 hours for women and for men over the age of 65

One alcohol drink is defined as about 12–15 grams of alcohol (ethanol), that is, 12 ounces of beer, 5 ounces of wine, or 1½ ounces of spirits (hard liquor, like whiskey or vodka).

Positive health effects of small or moderate alcohol consumption include reduce risk for:

- Coronary heart disease, by raising the levels of good cholesterol (HDL)
- Type 2 diabetes
- Alzheimer's disease
- Gallstones

Small-to-moderate amounts of alcohol, preferably wine during meals, may also contribute to longer life expectancy.

Drinking more than the low recommended levels of alcohol can cause serious and life-threatening health conditions, which include:

- Fatal motor vehicle accidents
- Brain damage, including premature dementia
- Weakening of the heart muscle
- Atrial fibrillation
- Stroke
- High blood pressure
- Fatty liver
- Alcoholic liver disease
- Cirrhosis of the liver
- Acute and chronic pancreatitis and pancreatic failure
- Pneumonia
- Tuberculosis
- Reduced ability to fight infections

Alcohol use during pregnancy is damaging to the fetus. Also, according to NIH, alcohol abuse can also cause several cancers, including cancer of the:

- Mouth
- Esophagus
- Throat
- Liver
- Breast

Avoid drug use

Most drugs can profoundly change the way we think and respond to external stimuli, leading to potentially life-threatening health risks like:

- Addiction
- Drugged driving, leading to accidents
- Infectious disease, like HIV/AIDS, hepatitis B and C, and other sexually transmitted infections and infections of the heart valves ("endocarditis").

Most drugs can also harm an unborn baby. Drug abuse is inconsistent with a healthy lifestyle. Drug abuse can shorten our life even more than obesity, diabetes, or heart disease. An individual in his or her teens is not too young to die from drug abuse. Also, even if death is avoided, drug abuse will lead to ill health and strained personal, work, and social relationships. If you abuse drugs, they will take over your life; you will not be able to keep a family, a job, or a relationship. Drug abuse takes away control and direction in our lives and makes continuing drug use its sole or major purpose. The following is drug-specific information for some of the common drugs, as presented by the National Institute on Drug Abuse, a branch of NIH (National Institutes of Health).

Marijuana

Marijuana (street names: "dope," "grass," "pot," "smoke," "weed," "hashish") works by releasing large amounts of dopamine in your brain, making you feeling a pleasant "high." This discussion is even more relevant today, as the use of recreational marijuana is legal in certain US states and is not considered a criminal offence in others. Its use has been linked to strokes and heart attacks along with a three times higher than the average risk for death due to very high blood pressure (data published by Yankey BA et al, in the *European Journal of Preventive Cardiology*, 2017). Marijuana impairs short-term memory and judgment, adversely affects performance in school or at work, and can make driving dangerous. It has a negative impact on the developing brain of adolescents and young adults, potentially reducing their ability to learn and think for many years to follow. Marijuana can be addictive and can make it easier for the user to progress to even more dangerous drugs. While "medical marijuana" is gaining acceptance in many states, it has not earned an FDA approval. In the long run it can also cause depression and anxiety. Smoked marijuana can cause respiratory illness in a way similar to smoking cigarettes. It can increase the heart rate and, if used during pregnancy, it can affect the embryo's brain. Withdrawal symptoms include irritability, difficulty sleeping, anxiety, and reduced appetite.

Cocaine

Cocaine (street names include, among others, "C," "candy," "Charlie," "crack," "snow") is a strongly addictive stimulant drug. It can be snorted, smoked, or injected. It has been used for thousands of years by people in South America, and in the early 1900s cocaine was an active ingredient in many tonics and elixirs and even in early Coca-Cola® products. Even today it is used for anesthesia in some eye and ear-nose-and-throat surgical procedures. In the short run, along with the desired effects of euphoria and increased energy and alertness, it can cause arteries to go to spasm, potentially leading to heart attacks and stroke, even if these arteries are free of any cholesterol plaque. It also increases the pulse rate and blood pressure and leads to irregular heart rhythms, headaches, sleeplessness and restlessness, anxiety, panic attacks, and violent behavior. In the long run, cocaine damages the nose and destroys the sense of smell, leads to loss of appetite and poor nutrition, pregnancy complications, infections, and death. If injected and needles are shared, it can cause HIV/AIDS, hepatitis B and C, and other infectious diseases. Infection of the inside of the heart valves can kill.

Heroin

Heroin (street names: "dope," "horse," "H," "smack," "white horse") is a highly addictive opioid (a close relative to morphine) drug that can be smoked, snorted, or injected. As its purity varies considerably, it is very easy to overdose, leading to slowing of the pulse and the respirations and potentially resulting in coma or even death. While it can make its user feel like he or she is on cloud nine, in reality, plays with the user's life. Beyond coma and death from overdose, heroin can kill through infections that affect the inner lining of the heart and its valves ("endocarditis"), through HIV/AIDS, hepatitis B and C, liver or kidney disease, and pneumonia. The entire "business" of heroin, while lethal for the user, keeps alive a robust and violent crime circle of production, manufacturing, and distribution. Beyond its direct unhealthy effects for the users, it plagues families and the workplace, entire sections of the society, at a cost of billions of dollars each year.

Methamphetamine

Methamphetamine (street names include "crank," "crystal," and "meth speed") is a strong and highly addictive stimulant. It increases wakefulness and physical activity and reduces appetite. It increases both pulse and breathing rate and can cause high blood pressure and irregular heartbeat. Its mental effects include anxiety, confusion, difficulty sleeping, mood swings, hallucinations, and violent behavior. It can destroy the teeth and causes itching and skin sores. It can cause serious problems in pregnancy. In the US, it is both a problem for the user and the society. It contributes to crime, unemployment, child neglect and/or abuse and costs more than 20 billion a year.

Obtain age and disease appropriate immunizations

Do not miss necessary immunizations and preventive tests.

Vaccines

Contrary to some popular beliefs, immunizations (vaccinations) do work and their serious side effects are rare. They protect not only the individuals that get vaccinated but the entire community, as they radically reduce the number of infected individuals. They are credited with eradicating small-pox, a true killer disease (last case occurred in Somalia in 1977) and eliminating other serious diseases in many countries (polio was eliminated in the US in 1979). Largely through vaccinations, polio, measles, mumps, and rubella are on the brink of eradication all over the world. Common immunizations include:

- Influenza (flu) vaccine
- Pneumococcal vaccine
- Herpes zoster vaccine
- Tetanus and diphtheria
- HPV early in life (adults younger than 26 years)

The Centers for Disease Control make the following recommendation regarding adult vaccination:

1. Pneumococcal vaccine

This vaccine reduces the chance of developing pneumococcal disease that can cause meningitis and pneumonia. It is recommended for:

- Anyone who is 65 or older
- Anyone between 19 and 65 years of age with asthma or who is a smoker

- Anyone between the ages of 2 and 65 with heart disease, lung disease, sickle cell disease, diabetes, alcoholism, cirrhosis, leaks of cerebrospinal fluid, or a cochlear implant
- Anyone between the ages of 2 and 65 with a condition that lowers resistance to infection, including lymphoma, leukemia, HIV or AIDS, kidney failure, a damaged or missing spleen, or organ transplant
- Anyone between the ages of 2 and 65 receiving a treatment that lowers resistance to infection, including radiation therapy, some cancer drugs, or long-term steroids
- Anyone living in a nursing home or long-term care facility

2. Human papillomavirus (HPV) vaccine

This vaccine protects against HPV, a virus that can cause genital cancer (cervical, vaginal, and vulvar) and genital warts. Beyond children, HPV vaccine is also recommended for young adults (men and women 26 years old or younger) who were not vaccinated as children.

3. Influenza (flu) vaccine

Seasonal influenza vaccination is recommended yearly for all adults. The vaccine protects against respiratory illness caused by influenza viruses. Because new strains of influenza appear frequently, the seasonal flu vaccine usually changes each year.

4. Tetanus/diphtheria and tetanus/diphtheria/pertussis booster vaccines

A combination vaccine against tetanus, diphtheria, and pertussis (whooping cough) is given in childhood in a series of shots called DTaP. Pregnant women are recommended to take the Tdap vaccine during the last trimester of each pregnancy in order to protect their baby. While routine boosters should be given every 10 years, this vaccine is also given to individuals who have suffered injuries or wounds that may have exposed them to tetanus bacteria.

5. Hepatitis A vaccine

Hepatitis A vaccines were added to the routine childhood immunizations in 2006 but are also recommended for adults who are at an increased risk for hepatitis A. This includes the following groups:

- Anyone traveling to developing countries
- Men who have sex with men
- Anyone who uses illegal drugs
- Anyone who works with non-human primates infected with hepatitis A or who works with hepatitis A in a research setting
- Anyone with chronic liver disease
- Anyone with clotting factor disorders

Also, this vaccination may be considered for food handlers because of their potential to transmit the virus to others.

6. Hepatitis B vaccine

Hepatitis B vaccines are recommended for:

- Anyone living with or having sex with a hepatitis B-infected person
- Anyone having sex with multiple partners
- Anyone seeking treatment for sexually transmitted diseases, HIV testing, or drug treatment
- Men who have sex with men
- Anyone who uses illegal drugs
- Anyone with a job that involves direct contact with human blood
- Anyone who has HIV
- Anyone with severe chronic kidney or liver disease
- Anyone who is a prisoner in a correctional facility
- Anyone who is traveling to a country where the virus is common

7. Measles, mumps, and rubella (MMR) vaccine

Adults who were born in the US after 1957 *may* need to receive booster shots or be revaccinated with MMR if they are:

- College students
- Health care workers
- Individuals traveling internationally

Also, women of childbearing age who want to become pregnant and have no evidence of immunity against rubella and individuals who have received several types of measles vaccine from 1963 to 1967 need to receive the MMR vaccine.

8. Chickenpox (varicella) vaccine

The vaccine is recommended for adults with no evidence of chickenpox immunity, like those born in the United States after 1980, health care workers, and pregnant women irrespective of their age.

9. Shingles (zoster) vaccine

This vaccine is recommended for individuals who are 60 years of age or older, even if they have reported a previous case of shingles.

10. Meningococcal vaccine

This vaccine is recommended for anyone who is:
- A member of the military
- An individual with damaged or removed spleen
- Doing research that exposes him/her to Neisseria meningitidis
- Traveling to a country where meningococcal disease is common
- Starting college and has not received a dose of the vaccine during the previous five years

Travel vaccine

Some vaccines may be required before you are allowed to enter a particular country or region like:
- Tropical South America or sub-Saharan Africa
- Certain developing countries

More information can be found on the Centers for Disease Control and Prevention's Traveler's Health website. In addition to vaccines, travel medicine centers can advise on prevention of malaria and certain types of infectious diarrhea.

Vitamins and supplements

Vitamins are small molecules that are necessary for life. But do we need to be taking them in the form of supplements? The *Dietary Guidelines for Americans* suggest that a healthy eating pattern through a balanced diet and, in the case of vitamin D, a few minutes of sun exposure a couple of times per week, should be more than enough to meet our body's requirements. There are, however, some occasions where vitamins should be taken as supplements. For example, the FDA points out that "the use of folic acid supplements by women of childbearing age who may become pregnant reduces the risk of some birth defects" and that "vitamin B12 is beneficial in people over age 50 who often have a reduced ability to absorb the naturally occurring forms of this vitamin." On the other hand, certain vitamins, when taken as supplements, can be harmful, like supplements containing vitamin A, E, or beta carotene. For most vitamins, however, the jury is still out and the available scientific evidence, as imperfect as it always has been, is so contradictory and confusing that it cannot give us a simple "Yes" or "No" when it comes to most vitamin supplements.

The supplement industry is huge. It is estimated that more than 36 billion USD are spent on vitamins and supplements in the US every year. And the China supplements market is rising fast, so there is a big global economy in regards to vitamins and supplements. And, scientific evidence notwithstanding, it is based on the perception, so prevalent among us consumers, that vitamins and supplements are good for our health.

While all vitamins taken in their natural form (that is, as part of the foods we eat—usually fruits and vegetables, fish, and some meats) are definitely beneficial, the same cannot be said when they are taken as supplements. Scientific research about the majority of vitamin supplements has yielded inconclusive, conflicting and contradictory results with no easy answers, either for the professionals or the consumers.

In the US, dietary supplements are not required by federal law to be tested for safety and effectiveness before they are marketed. Many of the claims about miraculous health benefits on the supplements label are overstated and, occasionally, even harmful ingredients have been found in the pills. The FDA, however, does require that supplement labels include a disclaimer about the health benefits the manufacturer claims that reads "... This statement has not been evaluated by the FDA. This product is not intended to diagnose, treat, cure, or prevent any disease."

So, in a nutshell, taking these supplements from reputable brands that are careful not to include any harmful ingredients can be good, bad, or have no effect at all (although not all scientists agree on all those points):

Recommended vitamins and supplements, proven or promising:
- Vitamin D – helps bone and artery health
- Vitamin B12 –good for people over 50
- Folic Acid – good for all women of childbearing age who might become pregnant
- Fish Oil – reduces triglycerides
- CoQ10 – supports heart and artery health and may reduce muscle aches due to statins

Questionable:
- Glucosamine/Chondroitin – help in knee arthritis is debated
- Vitamin C – evidence is conflicting in regards to cancer or heart disease prevention
- Resveratrol – may slow down aging and protect against Alzheimer's, but evidence is conflicting
- NAD – may slow down aging
- Vitamin B complex supplements – little evidence to support their use

Vitamins not to take:
- Vitamin A – touted as a potent antioxidant, protecting against cancer and heart disease. Studies have shown, however, that when vitamin A is taken as a supplement, bad things happen: more cases of bleeding strokes, prostate cancer, and lung cancer (among smokers) were noted.
- Beta carotene, a precursor of vitamin A – studies have found that beta carotene supplements may increase the risk of heart disease and cancer in people who smoke or drink heavily.

- Vitamin E – while a powerful antioxidant, studies have found that vitamin E supplements can be harmful for individuals suffering from cancer. Vitamin E may increase the risk of prostate cancer and can increase the risk of bleeding in people taking certain type of blood thinners. Most scientists do not recommend taking vitamin E supplements.

Screening Procedures

Screening tests aim to identify important diseases early, before symptoms develop. Popular screening tests and the conditions they are designed to detect include:
- Cholesterol and blood pressure, for prevention of artery and heart disease
- Mammograms and pap-tests, for early detection of breast and cervical cancer, respectively
- Colonoscopy and prostate exams, for early detection of colon and prostate cancer, respectively
- Skin exams, for early detection of melanoma

The thinking is that early identification/detection leads to better treatment and potential cures. Things are not always that simple:
- Identifying a slow-growing prostate cancer that would have never caused any problem to the individual (as many older men are more likely to die with prostate cancer than die of prostate cancer) may cause unnecessary anxiety, treatment, and harm without any benefit.
- Early identification of an aggressive breast cancer may not necessarily increase chances of survival.

On the other hand, there is very good evidence that early identification of:
- High blood pressure saves many lives and decreases strokes, heart attacks, and heart failure.
- Screening colonoscopies has also been proven to save lives by identifying colon and rectal cancer at early stages when they are more likely to be curable.

The most popular screening test are:

Blood pressure

Self monitoring your blood pressure through a reliable digital blood pressure cuff allows you to identify high blood pressure early, before it damages your arteries and your heart.

Consider that blood pressure measurement at the doctor's office usually overestimates your blood pressure (as the patient may be experiencing anxiety-whether consciously or unconsciously) and may lead to overdiagnosis and unnecessary treatment. Self-monitoring your BP (e.g., once a month if you are 30 or older or more frequently if you are obese, overweight, a smoker, or have prediabetes or diabetes) not only allows you early diagnosis of an important disease but also proves that you do care about your health, and this is huge! Beyond preventing heart disease and stroke, early diagnosis of high blood pressure helps protect your kidneys and eyes and reduce vascular dementia and aneurysms. Normal BP is below 120/80 mmHg. If your blood pressure is often above 140/90 mmHg, see your doctor; don't forget to bring together your home BP log and all the medicines, including over-the-counter, and supplements that you take.

LDL cholesterol

Best way: through your primary care provider. Although the current scientific recommendation is to check it once every five years, some providers check it routinely during an annual wellness visit. According to the current guidelines, if your LDL is above 190 mg/dl, you need to take medications to prevent artery disease. Individuals with already diagnosed heart disease, diabetes, kidney disease, stroke, or blockages in the leg arteries are usually placed on medications that lower LDL for life as a means of preventing worsening artery disease.

Blood sugar and A1c

Best way: through your primary care provider. Current recommendations suggest screening once every three years, especially after the age of 45.

In case of high blood pressure or high cholesterol (especially high tri-glycerides), screening must start earlier and be repeated on a yearly basis. A fasting blood sugar below 100 mg/dl or an A1c below 5.7% is considered normal. A fasting blood sugar of 100–125 or an A1c of 5.7–6.4% is considered prediabetes (meaning increased risk of developing diabetes in the future, especially if a first degree relative has type 2 diabetes). Values of 126 or higher (blood sugar) or 6.5% or higher (A1c) indicate full-blown diabetes.

TSH

Best way: through your primary care provider. Many providers routinely check TSH during wellness visits. The reason is that low thyroid conditions ("hypothyroidism"), while very important and common, frequently have subtle and nonspecific symptoms. Typically a patient may feel as though they are having "low energy," but don't we all? A high TSH implies low-thyroid state and calls for thyroid hormone supplementation. A low TSH is a less frequent finding and indicates high thyroid state, which also needs to be medically treated.

Creatinine

There are no routine recommendations for checking creatinine, a blood test that reflects kidney function. However, a high creatinine level can be an early sign of kidney disease (disease killer #9) and a common health problem among those who have high blood pressure or diabetes, smoke, or are overweight, are African-American, are over 50 years old, or take certain medications (NSAIDs like ibuprofen, naproxen, or diclofenac). Consider that a person can have as little as 10–20 percent of kidney function before experiencing any symptoms.

Screening for colon cancer

Starting at age 50, this truly life-saving and highly recommended screening should proceed in one of the following three ways:
- A stool specimen test for occult blood once a year
- Colonoscopy every 10 years

- Flexible sigmoidoscopy every five years plus stool tests every three years

A strong family history of colon cancer or polyps, history of inflammatory bowel disease (ulcerative colitis or Crohn's disease), or colon polyps implies more frequent testing and regular visits to your gastroenterologist.

Breast self-exam

Doctors' opinions on the value of breast self-exam differ, as there is no strong scientific evidence that it really saves lives. However, performing a breast self-exam once a month, at the very least, proves that you care about your health, and this is a truly winning attitude in the life-long marathon of wellness. The sooner after adolescence you start a breast self-examination, the better.

Mammograms

A mammogram is an x-ray picture of the breast. It is recommended that women between the age of 40 and 75 have a mammogram for early detection of breast cancer, every one to two years. Women with a first degree relative with breast cancer should start having mammograms at an age younger than the age of breast cancer diagnosis in their mother or sister. If you have other risk factors for breast cancer, your provider may recommend a mammogram, breast ultrasound, or MRI scan. Early detection of breast cancer with screening mammography leads to earlier treatment, possibly before cancer has spread. There is good scientific evidence that screening mammography can help reduce the number of deaths from breast cancer in women between the ages of 40 and 74.

Pelvic exam and Pap smear

Pap-test tells one of the most impressive success stories in medicine: according to the NIH, cervical cancer incidence and death rates in the US have declined by more than 60 percent between 1955 and 1992! Pap test (and HPV—human papillomavirus—testing) is recommended for all women between the ages of 21 and 65 years old, once every three years. After the age of 30, if the HPV test is negative, a Pap test is recommended only once every five years. If you have undergone hysterectomy with removal of the cervix and have no history of cervical cancer, you no longer need Pap tests. After age 65, those women who have not been diagnosed with cervical cancer or precancerous abnormalities on Pap smears can stop having Pap tests as long as they have had three negative tests within the previous 10 years, unless they have other risk factors.

Prostate cancer screening

Screenings for early diagnosis of prostate cancer among healthy men usually include a direct examination of the prostate through digital rectal exam (DRE) and blood test (PSA, for "prostate specific antigen"). As we have already mentioned, what makes prostate screening controversial is that a slow growing cancer that was never going to cause any real symptoms may be identified early through screening, leading to overdiagnosis and overtreatment, accompanied by much anxiety, cost, and potentially dangerous medical procedures. Most men are destined to have some cancer cells by the time they die, but whether that condition results in any health problems is another story. So, it should come as no surprise that government guidelines recommend against the routine use of the PSA test. The American Cancer Society advises men to talk with their doctor, beginning at age 50 for the average-risk person (40–45 years for those with a family history of prostate cancer or African Americans), about the potential risks and benefits of the PSA testing.

Lung cancer screening

The USPSTF (US Preventive Services Task Force) recommends annual screening for lung cancer with low-dose computed tomography (a type of CAT scan) for current or former (who quit in the past 15 years) smokers between the ages of 55 and 80 years, provided that they have smoked heavily and long enough so as to have a 30 pack-year (e.g., one pack per day for 30 years, half a pack per day for 60 years or two packs per day for 15 years) smoking history.

Skin cancer screening

The most dangerous form of skin cancer is melanoma. It is more common in men than in women, and the risk increases with age. The American Cancer Society and the American Academy of Dermatology recommend regular skin self-exams to check for any changes in marks on your skin including shape, color, and size. A skin exam by a dermatologist or other health professional should be part of a routine checkup. Treatments for skin cancer are more effective, and the condition is less disfiguring when it's found early.

Screening for sexually transmitted infections

Chlamydia and gonorrhea are the #2 and #4 most common sexually trans-mitted diseases in the US (#1 is HPV, usually diagnosed during a Pap smear or from genital warts). Women up to the age of 25 (or older, if at high risk) should be screened for chlamydia and gonorrhea. A pelvic exam can pro-duce not only a Pap smear but also samples for diagnosis of chlamydia and gonorrhea. A Pap test can be done during a pelvic exam, but not all pelvic exams include a Pap test. An HPV test can be done on the same sample of cells collected from the Pap test.

Eye Screening for Glaucoma

Eye tests for glaucoma are based on age and personal risk:
- Under 40: Every 2–4 years
- 40-54: Every 1–3 years
- 55-64: Every 1–2 years
- 65 up: Every 6–12 months

Talk with your doctor about earlier, more frequent screening if you fall in a high risk group, including African-Americans, those with a family history of glaucoma, previous eye injury, or use of steroid medications.

Dental exam

See your dentist once or twice a year for an exam and cleaning. But do not consider a periodic dental exam to be a substitute for flossing daily or brushing your teeth two times a day!

Screening for depression

Depression is common, painful, and potentially life-threatening. It is among the leading causes of disability in people older than 15. As most patients with depression will go to their primary care provider rather than a psychiatrist, it is important that, during wellness visits, screening for depression takes place. The screening is simple and is usually done through a standardized questionnaire; the process is quick, low-cost, low-risk, and efficient. The USPSTF (US Preventive Services Task Force) recommends screening for depression, as it found adequate evidence that depression screening (along with adequate support systems and treatment with second-generation antidepressants or psychotherapy, as indicated) reduces suffering and disability at relatively low cost and low-to-moderate risk.

Screening for osteoporosis

Osteoporosis makes bones weak and brittle and fractures, especially of the hip and spine, more common. Osteoporosis is a common condition: approximately one in two women and up to one in four men age 50 are considered as having osteoporosis. By current scientific recommendations, women over the age of 64 should undergo a bone density test ("DEXA" scan).

Preventing sexually transmitted infections through safe sex

Chlamydia, HPV (human papillomavirus), gonorrhea, HIV/AIDS, syphilis, and hepatitis B and C are major sexually transmitted infections (STIs). Many STIs primarily affect the reproductive organs, resulting in infection, sores, pain, or an unusual discharge. Other STIs can also affect the body's immune system or other organs. To prevent those diseases, be fully aware of your partner's sexual history and any diseases they may have. With a new partner, it is best for both of you to get checked for STIs. Always use protection during sex, such as condoms, and know how to use them properly. Since transmission of infected bodily fluids can pass on STIs, don't share needles.

Have a "won't give up" attitude

Related to living for a purpose a "won't give up attitude" is a necessary element of a healthy lifestyle. Adversity happens. Success and failure come in never-ending cycles. Problems and stress are a permanent feature of life. If life were a track and field event, it would be a hybrid of marathon with hurdles and a decathlon. Life is not easy as it is; aging diminishes our initial health capital, making matters even more challenging. However, a "won't give up" attitude, coupled with a healthy dose of confidence and self-esteem, daily discipline regarding healthy diet and adequate physical activity, adequate sleep, fulfillment at work, and never accepting the stereotypical "getting older means slowing down" will help you achieve your life goals. You will achieve not only a longer lifespan but a longer healthspan (how many years you live in good health) too.

So, don't give up if:
- A person close to you disappoints or betrays you
- If a loved one dies or becomes sick
- If your boss is not appreciative of your performance and sacrifices at work
- If your financial investments fail
- If you gain back some of the weight you so painfully and with so many deprivations managed to lose
- If you eat a big ice cream or a milk chocolate bar
- If you drank four beers with your friends over the weekend and woke up with a terrible hangover
- If you didn't exercise for a whole week

You fall, but you will rise again. This is human nature. This is part of how our bodies, souls, and minds function. Accept it as a norm, stand up again and again, and keep fighting. In the long run, over years and decades, this "won't give up" attitude will make you a big winner. You will look back to the adversity and disappointments of the past with the smile of tranquil satisfaction, success, and experience of a long and hard-fought struggle. If you give up on life, life returns the favor quickly and gives up on you.

Have a rich social life

This is especially important for individuals older than 65 years of age or retirees. Staying at home the entire day without a purpose and spending hours in front of TV will quickly make you depressed and senile. Your muscles will atrophy, and very quickly you will start seeing no purpose in life. Have a friend or a relative with whom you visit frequently and have something to discuss—a book, a trip, a memory.

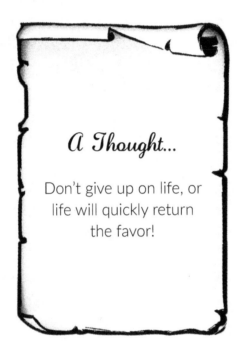

A Thought...

Don't give up on life, or life will quickly return the favor!

Live for a reason and give meaning to your life, every day

Whether it is serving God or your country, a culture or an idea, helping your family or your kids, learning a musical instrument or a foreign language, traveling, or whether it is an art, a sport, or a hobby, having always something to live for is instrumental in overcoming adversity. Stress and adversity are almost permanent parts of life; they must be considered as a given. It is only their timing, frequency, intensity, and specific nature that is uncertain. Adversity has many faces; it can come as an illness or debility, impossible stress at work, financial difficulty, litigation, or even even issues with loved ones. Having a "rock" to hold on to during these times is essential. How else can we keep persevering in overcoming adversity and finding meaning by doing so, especially as we are getting older? Without having a purpose or meaning in life, aging alone can be plenty to destabilize you, make you depressed, and make you feel as if life is no longer worth fighting for. Once you start feeling this way, the game is over, unless somebody or something can drag you out of these morbid thoughts fast! Once you no longer believe in life, it is easier for your cells to turn to cancer, your arteries to form clots, and germs and infections to overwhelm you. Depression alone can kill you, indirectly (through drugs and alcohol) or directly (by committing suicide). If you think you may be depressed, talk to your doctor.

It is unrealistic to expect to face life's problems day in and day out without having a deep entrenched, strong reason to live for.

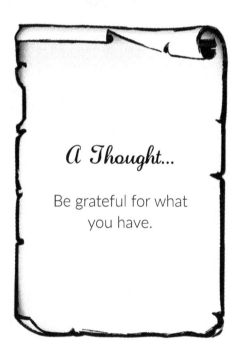

A Thought...

Be grateful for what
you have.

A major cause of the unnatural stress that destroys our health and our lives is wanting so many more things that we do not need or cannot have. And this holds true for everybody, even the richest among us. Once a person has enough money in the bank and a good home and car, next may be wanting an even larger and more luxurious home, expensive trips, a yacht, a private jet, a private island, an even bigger business and more market share. The pursuit for more is endless. Now, there are some things we do consider essential: food, shelter, electricity, internet access. And, first and foremost, sound health and satisfying personal relationships. Once those needs are met, the rest must be considered optional and not an absolute necessity.

Feeling grateful for what we have—health, personal relationships, essential material needs—is a very good way to start our everyday life journey. If we lack this feeling of gratefulness for what we already have, we will never be happy, no matter what we achieve. And this morbid psychology of greediness that breeds unhappiness will spill into our biology, into the workings of our body's organs, all the way into our cells. Then, before we know it, there is an unstable cholesterol plaque, a clot, a cancer cell, depression, alcohol, drugs, destroyed relationships, and an ugly end.

Chapter 6 Questions

1. You take painkillers for arthritis. You have tried several over the years and found out that they all work well, as long as you take them daily. You take the dose of this medications that your doctor has prescribed. Out of the following medications, which one is the safest to take in the long run?
   - Tylenol
   - Motrin
   - Vicodin
   - Ibuprofen
   - Diclofenac

2. How many hours are you supposed to sleep every day?

3. Are 30 minutes of walking, five days a week enough to qualify as a healthy lifestyle?

4. You are a 70-year-old woman who recently retired and lives alone. Which of the following interventions or behaviors can help you live a long, healthy life?
   a. Visiting friends frequently
   b. Eating healthy
   c. Not smoking
   d. Not drinking more than one alcoholic beverage per day
   e. All of the above
   f. Only b, c, and d

5. Is recreational marijuana safe?

6. What immunizations are essential for individuals over the age of 65?

Chapter 7

THE VISION: LIVING HEALTHY 360 DEGREES

"Early to bed and early to rise, makes a man healthy, wealthy and wise"
—Benjamin Franklin

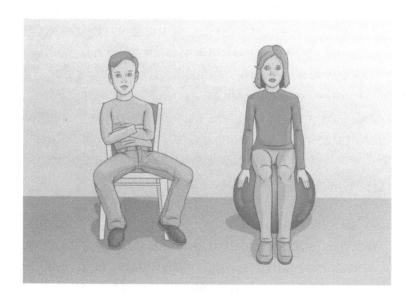

Is the obesity-diabetes-artery disease epidemic invincible? Is it our destiny, as Americans, to go down in a swirl of belly fat, added sugars, incessant sitting, and irresponsible finances? Since the late 1970s—when obesity rates took off—there hasn't been much to be optimistic about in terms of defeating the epidemic. Something very substantial in the way we live, eat, drink, work, play, sleep, and interact with each other has got to change.

In previous chapters we have outlined how the epidemic concerns us all, not only those who are obese or diabetic. Acknowledging the interconnectedness of all of us—through our health and our finances—establishes the social aspect of the epidemic. The dependence of the epidemic on both social and individual factors suggests that all of us bear the responsibility for finding and implementing a viable and lasting solution: not only you and me as individuals but also all of us as a community; not only you and me as employees but also our employers. And as the epidemic hinges on lifestyle, we must re-engineer almost every aspect of human life as we know it: from what and how much we eat and drink to the ways we live, work, move, shop, play, and sleep. Hopes that a miracle drug or a medical procedure will stop obesity and diabetes are unrealistic. Pills and procedures can only provide management (not cures!) of obesity-related disorders (including type 2 diabetes, high blood pressure, and others) and cannot prevent obesity and diabetes in the first place; only a healthy lifestyle can.

And it takes two to tango: to turn the tide of the epidemic through healthier lifestyles, **society** must create the appropriate opportunities (at school and the workplace) and **individuals** must take advantage of those opportunities (and, additionally, create an equally healthy environment at home). And while hospitals or doctors cannot prevent obesity, our primary care providers do play a very important role by raising the red flag when our waistlines increase or our blood pressure, LDL cholesterol, or A1c start trending upwards. Re-engineering our relation with both our primary care providers and medical specialists is actually part of our fight against the epidemic, by halting the advance of obesity, high blood pressure, and diabetes and preventing their deadly complications.

Necessity and a harsh life helped the Paleo man achieve great fitness and, if lucky enough to escape starvation, consume a healthy diet. On the other hand, lack of necessity for hard physical work (nowadays an employee can be 100 percent productive—and handsomely paid—in spite of being 100 percent sedentary!) and the availability of virtually unlimited quantities of health-damaging added sugars and salt have led us astray. This "progress" has made us obese and diabetic in numbers never seen before in the history of mankind.

We have reached a point in our evolution as humans that we **must** change (now and forever)
- The way we use our many artifacts (cars and chairs, computers and smartphones)
- The ways we produce and process food.

We must put purpose and survival over comfort and "coolness," tame our demands for pleasure and "fun," and make our gadgets and our activities work to our advantage and not to our destruction. For example, wearables like Fitbit hold great promise for helping us self-monitor our health, as they already allow us to count how many steps we take in a day. It is very likely that, in the near future, wearables will allow us to monitor our blood pressure (BP) and enable us to present our doctor with hundreds of BP measurements that will make diagnosis easier.

The obesity-diabetes-artery disease epidemic is acutely pressing us, and time is running out: even if we change today, good results will take years and decades to achieve; consider that it took half a century to win over the tobacco addiction and dramatically reduce smoking rates from a 42% (in the mid 60s) to only 15% today. Winning over the obesity-diabetes-artery disease epidemic is likely to be more difficult and take even longer, but if we are determined, it can be done.

I have spent over three decades as a physician sitting across patients with obesity or type 2 diabetes, heart attacks, atrial fibrillation, heart failure, or stroke. Here are some of the things I learned along the way:
- People usually gain weight as they age. The older we get, the more difficult it is to get rid of it and keep it off. When I talk to my patients

about diet and exercise, I almost take for granted that very few will be able to lose weight and keep it off in the long run.

- Weight gain doesn't have to do only with genes and age or with our motivation about healthy eating and moving. It has also to do with the responsibilities, whether assigned or self-imposed, at work, at school, or at home. When our job can be done well while we are comfortably seated, why choose moving our bodies or using our muscles?
- Stress is constantly present in our lives. For so many of us there are hardly any long stress-free periods. Therefore, we almost never have stress-free time to quit smoking or try to lose weight.
- People are much more concerned about side effects of medications that treat high blood pressure or cholesterol than about the side effects of high blood pressure or abnormal cholesterol (like stroke, heart attacks, heart failure, atrial fibrillation, or sudden death).
- There are challenges after one survives a heart attack or is paralyzed after a stroke.

Humans are not robots and therefore we cannot:

- Count and track calories, carbs, and saturated fats every day for all our meals and snacks
- Always refuse a tasty treat just because it gets our saturated fat allowance over the 10% recommended daily limit
- Commit to a long-term lifestyle that makes our everyday life miserable, just because it promises a longer (still miserable) life

So, in this chapter I present a realistic plan for a long-term, all out war against the obesity-diabetes-artery disease epidemic; my vision as to what has to change in the way we live, work, eat, drink, play, and sleep. My suggestions are straightforward and palatable. We can implement them for the rest of our lives and persuade our spouses, kids, parents, friends, and co-workers to do the same. The result? We can make obesity and diabetes as rare as they were 50 years ago:

- Obesity was affecting less than 15% of the adult US population; today, 37% of Americans are obese
- Diabetes rate was then less than 2%; today, it is almost 10%

My strategy

The goal is to defeat the epidemic while we maintain a comfortable way of living—we keep electricity and the Internet, our cars, computers, and smartphones. And although every aspect of our life should change, my strategy focuses on **four key fronts**:

- School
- Workplace
- Home
- Society and the WellPals

On these fronts there are **four main lifestyle choices** to tackle on a daily basis:

- Diet
- Physical Activities
- Not smoking
- Other

Let's discuss, first, the lifestyle choices.

1. Diet

Food should provide:

- Energy
- Protein
- Good Fats (omega-3 and MUFAs, see Chapter 6)
- Vitamins
- Antioxidants
- Fiber
- Potassium
- Pleasure

What we should try to avoid:

- **Added Sugars** (limit them to about 30 g a day for women and 40 g a day for men) are simple sugars that are added to food during preparation or processing. Naturally occurring simple sugars are found in fruits, vegetables, milk, and honey.

- **Salt** (limit it to 1.5–2.3 g per day. American Heart Association recommends limiting sodium to 1.5 g a day whereas FDA recommends limiting sodium to 2.3 g per day).
- **Saturated Fats** (ideally no more than 20–25 g a day for women and 25–30 g a day for men). However—and this is a critical point of my vision—eliminating added sugars is more important than controlling saturated fat.

How do added sugars work in our bodies?

Once they reach our taste buds and send pleasure signals left and right in the reward center of our brain, we can't stop having them. Most of us have experienced this during our lifetime: after we start eating ice cream, donuts, candies, or chocolate, we just can't stop! We feel powerless! At the same time, we know too well how bad this is for our waistlines and our health.

The case with saturated fats is different: animal fats (and the protein that comes along with them) have a much more pronounced satiety effect than sugars, especially when accompanied by fiber in the form of vegetables (how often have you tried donuts with tomatoes, versus red meat with tomatoes). We love melted cheese and red meat, but there is a point when we feel full and stop eating. It is difficult to reach this point while savoring ice cream, donuts, candies, or chocolate. Another important issue with added sugars is that they cause our insulin to spike (stressing our poor beta pancreas cells in the way) and, in less than two hours after a carb-rich meal, we get a mild hypoglycemia, experience hunger pangs, and start eating all over again!

Remember though, that we expect some pleasure out of eating. If foods are devoid of pleasure, we cannot stick to them in the long run. Consider, for example, how much more liberal than the American Heart Association and Dash diet the Paleo and Atkins diets are (they allow for much more saturated fat).

2. Physical Activities should include daily:

- **Endurance**: Two to four hours of light-to-moderate-intensity aerobic activities (cardio). Your goal should be to burn calories, maintain a healthy weight, preserve muscle mass, feel happier and more energetic, and reduce dementia. You do not have to run on the treadmill or use the stepper for two to four hours. **All you need to do is simply moving around for two to four hours a day**. If you have completed 15,000–20,000 steps taking care of your usual household chores or duties at work, you are done!

- **Strength**: Five to ten minutes a day of light to moderate strengthening (lifting weights or using elastic bands). Your goal: keep your muscles strong, as aging makes us lose muscle. This muscle loss slows down our metabolism, and it makes it easier to gain weight (fat) and more difficult to lose it. In addition, muscle wasting makes daily activities more challenging. In people in their 60s and 70s who have lost leg muscle, their legs feel so heavy that they walk slowly and often lose their balance. Actually, the older we get, the more time we have to invest to exercise.
- **Flexibility**: 10 to 20 minutes a day of stretching. Your goal: keep your muscles flexible and prevent muscle injuries. As a result, you will be able to perform your daily tasks better and easier, without injuring yourself (bending down to tie a shoe, walking upstairs, picking your kid up).
- **Balance**: 5 to 10 minutes a day. Your goal: avoid falls later in life. Falls can be devastating.

How long should we spend sitting?

We should limit total sitting time to six hours a day (including sitting at work, at home, during meals and during commuting). Also, we should stand up and stretch for a few seconds every 20 minutes.

3. No smoking

- No tobacco
- No vapor
- No hookah
- No marijuana

4. Other important issues

- Sleeping for seven to nine hours

- Avoiding third shift
- Limiting work to 55 hours per week
- Avoiding stress that is carried over from one day to the next
- Knowing our "numbers" (blood pressure, LDL, waist circumference, A1c, and blood sugar; see Chapter 6)

Now, **let's apply the lifestyle choices to the four main fronts** where the epidemic will be fought.

1. School

School is uniquely positioned to affect the habits and lifestyles of children and adolescents, not only during the formative school years but also for the rest of their lives. Therefore, school is instrumental in setting the foundations for a healthy lifestyle during adulthood. The current state of the obesity epidemic is dire and is getting worse. School-age students are destined to become obese adults in greater numbers than ever before. A new study found that out of today's children, almost 6 out of 10 will be obese by the age of 35 (compared to 3 out of 10 today); in other words, today's schools produce obese individuals at almost twice the rate they did just 20 years ago.

Faced with the acute threat of an obese and diabetic society, we need a paradigm shift: **school curriculum can no longer take priority over children's health**. Academic achievement in science and mathematics must take a second place, behind health achievements. Any competitive advantage of a more educated future workforce will be annihilated by the disadvantages of a future sick, obese, and diabetic workforce.

To adjust to the challenges of the epidemic in the 21st century, schools should:
- Limit the availability of added sugars (less than 10 g per day).
- Limit the availability of salt (less than 1 g per day).
- Not offer cold cuts or deep fried foods.
- Promote only water (including flavored, unsweetened water), fruits, vegetables, low-fat dairy, legumes, eggs, nuts, and seeds in their cafeterias. No sugary beverages, candies, cakes, ice cream, or sweets should be available (in the cafeteria or in vending machines).

- Limit sitting to no more than two hours per day, preferably on exercise balls and on the ground.
- Limit screen time to no more than 1.5 hours per day.
- Be equipped with standing desks that students can use for up to two hours a day.
- Offer walking classes (peripatetic, museum-style or headphone-based).
- Promote hybrid classes where children engage in learning in various physically active ways: sitting on exercise balls or on the ground, standing, and walking.
- Train students in the cafeteria on how to prepare their own simple, healthy meals from fresh ingredients. Young kids can be very effective in passing on this type of knowledge to their parents.
- Consider including the biology of type 2 diabetes and atherothrombosis (cholesterol plaque and blood clotting) in the Biology curriculum. Along with learning about photosynthesis, it will greatly benefit the students to learn how to prevent diabetes from destroying their adult lives.
- Have teachers trained (see WellPals) in the essentials of the obesity-diabetes-artery disease epidemic so they can identify students at risk for obesity or sedentary behavior, warn their parents, and suggest a visit to the child's pediatrician.

2. Workplace

For the average working American who spends eight hours at work and one hour commuting, there are not enough hours in the day to practice a healthy lifestyle, unless the opportunity is provided for a minimum of two hours of light-to-moderate physical activity at work. I will prove this point in the **let's do the numbers** section. I don't mean that you have to spend two hours in the gym at work but, rather, that your job is organized in such a way that it naturally involves a couple of hours of moving around and using your muscles. This is my vision for re-engineering the workplace, physically and functionally—and all this without any negative impact on productivity. It will take a team of professionals to give a new meaning to the term "workplace ergonomics," which includes not only avoiding hurting yourself from repetitive movements but also promoting your wellness and disease prevention.

A workplace that supports a healthy lifestyle should:
- Restrict sitting to four hours or less per working day
- Provide standing desks or exercise balls as an alternative to sitting
- Include movement (light-to-moderate physical activity) for at least two hours per day
- Interrupt sitting at least every 20 minutes for brief stand ups and stretches
- Allow for at least seven hours of sleep
- Restrict third shift
- Aim at finishing the workload of the day at the end of the physical day (lingering, unlimited responsibilities contribute to unnatural stress)
- Hold standing or treadmill meetings and conferences
- Educate employees about early signs and late complications of obesity, sedentary behavior, and unhealthy diet through wellness workshops

The workplace cafeteria should:
- Limit added sugars to 20 g a day
- Limit salt to 1.5 g per day
- Offer fruits, vegetables, good fats (olive oil, fish, nuts, seeds), lean meat, low-fat dairy, and eggs at affordable prices

Let's do the numbers!

The purpose of this paragraph is to show that, for the average working American, there are not enough hours in the day to allow for daily healthy lifestyle. As our current culture considers acceptable to work for 8 to 12 hours a day, five days a week, we need to examine whether the time left can accommodate the activities that are necessary for a healthy lifestyle, like:
- Seven to nine hours of sleep
- Enough time to exercise: two to four hours of physical activities at home or in the gym, after or before work

The average working American spends
- 9.5 hours at work
- One hour commuting to and from work

- 4.5 hours for household activities, eating and drinking, caring for others, and other "down time" (talking to your spouse and kids, taking a shower, bathroom time)
- About 30 minutes for personal time
- About one hour trying to fall asleep

Now, let's do the math:
- 9–13 hours of sleep and physical activities/exercise
- 16.5 hours for work, commuting, household activities, etc.

Total: 25.5–27.5 hours per 24-hour day: not enough hours in the day, resulting in **a time deficit of about 2-3 hours a day**

So, **for the average working American, there is not enough time in the day to live healthy.** No wonder, then, we are dealing with a raging obesity-diabetes-artery disease epidemic!

And you need to consider that these calculations represent a best-case scenario under ideal assumptions like:
- Availability of home exercise equipment, like a home treadmill, stationary bike, elliptical, and/or weights, or zero commuting time between home and the gym
- Ideal motivation and discipline so that, once other necessary activities are completed, there is no down time between activities (behaving almost like a robot, at times, so that not even a second goes wasted)

This leaves us with two viable options:
1. We reduce daily working time by about two hours a day AND persuade ourselves to start exercising as soon as work is over and without any delays
2. We accommodate physical activity during working hours

For a variety of reasons, option #2 appears more feasible and desirable. So, what does this mean? It means that **the workplace needs to be transformed** into a place where we not only work but we are also given the opportunity to routinely practice a healthy lifestyle (being physically active and follow a healthy diet) and, altogether, we behave in ways that combine enhanced productivity and healthy living.

Transforming the workplace into a place of healthy living with opportunities for physical activities and healthy diet is not one of the things that "can't be done." Adding physical activities during the work routine is not like cancelling gravity or moving time back. This transformation of the workplace is entirely doable, but it is not a "slam dunk"; it will take a significant change in the way both employees, employers, and customers view the workplace. It will take input from a team of professionals from diverse disciplines, like occupational medicine, physiotherapy, psychology, human factors, and ergonomics. It will also take sincere, coordinated, and cooperating efforts from all stakeholders like:
- Employers
- Regulators and policymakers
- Employees
- Customers, including both other employees or corporations and individuals who are not officially employed

During our workday, we should be given the opportunity for and be encouraged to take advantage of:
- At least two hours of low-to-moderate pace cardio activities, not only at the gym but also seamlessly incorporated into the work routine
- Limiting sitting time to no more than four hours
- Non-sitting working arrangements, like standing desks, must become available
- Eating healthy at work, including healthy lunch and healthy snacks
- Learning about wellness and disease prevention, including help from nurses or other medical professionals so that we become aware of "our numbers" like blood sugar, LDL cholesterol, and blood pressure
- Learning what a healthy lifestyle consists of and what the long-term complications of high blood pressure, abnormal cholesterol, prediabetes and diabetes, and artery disease are, through employer-sponsored health fairs

Finally, all these conditions should be applied **without compromising productivity**; actually, keeping employees happy, healthy, and active should improve productivity. Any other attempts to combine healthy workplace living with productive employment are hypocritical and destined to fail. As we have proven earlier in this chapter, unless we practice a healthy workplace lifestyle, leisure time exercise outside the workplace is not enough to cancel out 10 hours of sitting at work. And without a couple of hours of movement of any kind at work, there are not enough hours in the day to live healthy!

3. Home

Along with winding down after a long day at work and spending some quality time with family and friends, home activities should also include elements of wellness and prevention and provide time for:

Cooking meals from fresh ingredients (with lots of vegetables and up to 3–4 portions of fresh fruits, olive oil, fish or other lean protein, seeds, and nuts) and do what you have to do so that by the end of the day you have accomplished:

- At least two hours of light-to-moderate intensity aerobic activities or at least 15,000 steps in a day
- 5–10 minutes of resistance (strengthening) exercises,
- 5–10 minutes of balance exercises
- 10–20 minutes of stretching

If the above physical activities have already been completed at work, you are off the hook for the evening. Still, don't forget that total sitting time for the day (including work, commuting and at home) should be restricted to six hours.

For those who work at home, please refer to the **Workplace** section.

4. Community and WellPals: a case for community health activism

Knowledge is power. And knowledge about how belly fat leads to diabetes and heart attacks, how artery disease may work underground for decades before it hits swiftly and deadly, and how to best work with our primary care providers is necessary for defeating the epidemic. And while the Internet offers information, it does not offer knowledge, as it cannot provide structure or context. What about if the advice you are looking for, with structure and context, comes from someone you know and trust? Over my years as a practicing physician, I have been most impressed by how often people trust their friends and family with advice regarding health-related matters. And there are several reasons to support such a behavior:

- Friends and family (at least, some of them) have earned your trust over many, many years.
- They can listen to you without hurrying you up,
- There are no co-pays, no deductibles, and no long waiting times, and there is no cold and unfriendly hospital or clinic waiting environment.
- They may come up with a persuasive argument to have you see your doctor when you need to, even if you don't want to.

Have you heard of WellPals?

WellPals will consist of a friendly army of knowledgeable volunteers who will become the first line of defense against the obesity-diabetes-artery disease epidemic. They will be providing guidance and support to their family members, friends, and coworkers. They will be trained in a way similar to the way non-health care professionals learn how to perform CPR. They will know a thing or two about healthy lifestyle and will act as a very approachable liaison between medicine and the common man. And, as they grow in numbers and achieve a critical mass, they will be able to defeat the epidemic!

Over my years in practice I have been amazed by how often patients, when confronted with questions about their health, followed the advice of individuals who are non-professionals but familiar to them, like friends, members of their family, or coworkers. Advice from these friends—about, for example, whether to use or not medications for high blood pressure or cholesterol—is commonplace, and patients are, at times, more likely to heed a friend's suggestion than a doctor's recommendation. While I have practiced medicine in countries with strikingly different cultures, this phenomenon of following the medical advice of non-medical friends is surprisingly similar.

One of the most astonishing such instances that I personally experienced happened eight years ago when I was operating a cath lab in the southern Mediterranean island of Crete. A cath lab is a laboratory equipped with advanced technology for treating heart emergencies, like heart attacks. One Saturday morning, a 42-year-old shepherd from one of the mountainous villages started experiencing chest pain. He had to take care of some business in the city where my lab was and rode a taxi. The taxi driver was a close friend, and the shepherd mentioned his symptom of chest discomfort. The taxi driver listened carefully and told him not to worry. "Take some antacids, eat lightly for a day or two, and you will be just fine," he said.

As the man arrived in the city, his pain intensified and he talked to an aunt of his who was a breast cancer survivor and was more familiar with symptoms, diseases, doctors, and hospitals. She told him to go immediately to the hospital. The shepherd listened to his aunt and came to our hospital where an ECG showed that he was actually having a heart attack. We took him immediately to the cath lab, took pictures of his heart arteries, and put two stents in the main artery that was clogged and was threatening his life. The procedure did not present any unusual difficulties, considering that the cholesterol plaques and the clot could have easily taken his life. He responded very well to the treatment and suffered such minimal heart damage that it was hardly visible on an ultrasound of his heart the day after. Within 72 hours from his admission, he walked out of the hospital in pretty good condition, pain-free, and with an excellent outlook for the future.

When I asked him why he did not seek medical attention once he started having chest pain, his answer startled me: "The taxi driver, who is one of my best friends, told me not to worry; this man really cares for me. He is a person I know and trust!" This patient chose to follow, at least initially, the advice of a trusted friend over seeking the advice of a medical professional. He was lucky that his aunt—although not a medical professional herself—was more familiar with symptoms and gave him life-saving advice.

Her advice was the single most important element that saved his life. The critical link in the "chain of survival"- deciding to seek medical advice, being evaluated at a medical facility, being diagnosed as having a heart attack, being rushed to the cath lab, and finally receiving two stents in his main heart artery so that his heart attack was stopped and his life saved—was his aunt's recommendation to go to the hospital. The procedural events and details, although technically complex, are frequently a "routine" for trained medical professionals. The aunt's advice was more critical in saving this person's life than the high-tech medical procedure. And this patient is not alone in making decisions by listening to people he knew and trusted, irrespective of their medical qualifications. The phenomenon of following a trusted friend's advice over a doctor's recommendation is strong and widespread; hence my vision for the WellPals.

Who are the WellPals, and what can they do?

These "knowledge agents" will be laypeople, not health professionals, but they will be motivated, intelligent, enthusiastic, and willing to learn the basic facts about obesity, type 2 diabetes, high blood pressure, high LDL cholesterol, stroke, and heart disease. They will not need to learn all the biology details that doctors and nurses do. A WellPal will be **a person you already know and trust and with whom you feel comfortable**. When you open up to a WellPal, there will be no apprehension, no deductibles, and no co-pays.

It is a common scenario that, when a person feels unwell and must seek medical attention, but neither the situation is acute nor the suffering unbearable, one may hesitate and never take this first most difficult and critical step: to decide to go and see a physician. Entangled in a complex, fuzzy net of fear of an unfavorable diagnosis and what this may mean for his/her life, this person may start, often subconsciously, denying the problem and thinking of a million excuses for not going to the doctor: the need to take time off work, long waiting at the doctor's office, deductibles, co-pays, need for tests, needles, pain, and blood. It is so much easier to open up to a friend, a WellPal, and, supported by the WellPal's friendly suggestion, overcome those fears and inhibitions and decide to go and see the doctor.

Therefore, a **WellPal** is a friend, a coworker, or a member of your family. He or she is not a doctor or a nurse, but functions somewhat like non-professionals who are trained and certified to perform CPR (to deliver chest compression and even use a public defibrillator, an AED, to shock a dying heart out of its dangerous rhythm and back into life). In contrast to individuals trained to perform CPR, WellPals will receive training (and certification) to help guide people in the community to make the right decisions about prevention, wellness, and obesity-related diseases early, before a deadly disease strikes. Through their training, they will be able to, for example, advise you to talk to your child's pediatrician if there are early signs of obesity or the child appears to be too sedentary, to quit smoking or quit using hookah or vapor, to see your doctor when you were not going to (in spite of serious warning signs), to not use your cell phone while driving, to comply with treatment of high blood pressure when you were not going to and to understand what is happening (and going to happen) to your arteries when your LDL is 200 or your A1c is 8% and you act as if there is nothing wrong. WellPals will not replace doctors and nurses but will:

- Direct their friends to their health care providers when early signs appear
- Spread the message of wellness and prevention to the entire community
- Explain, in layman's terms, why abdominal fat, long hours of sitting, sugars, inadequate sleep, or excessive stress destroy our metabolisms
- Explain how an abnormal metabolism targets our arteries and puts us in the path of developing heart attacks, stroke, or sudden death
- Explain the effects of aging on our bodies
- Inform their friends about the risk factors for Alzheimer's and diabetes
- Suggest the use of a nutritionist and a personal trainer
- Encourage their friends to get flu shots and other immunizations
- Inform them about the benefit of screening procedures like mammograms and colonoscopies
- Teach their friends how to organize their own medical records
- Coach their friends on how to act and what to say and ask when they see their health care providers, so that they make the most out of their doctor's appointments

WellPals will fill the ranks of educators and policy makers, at the local, state, and federal level. Some of them will sit on school boards, be elected mayors, and participate in the local, state, and federal government, not to mention becoming presidents, first ladies, or cabinet members.

WellPals, while knowledgeable and certified in the area of obesity-and-diabetes-related diseases, are not health professionals. They are people like you and operate during casual social contacts; they are your trusted friend, your coworker, a member of your family. You interact with them during your daily activities. WellPals are in such great numbers in the community, that the chances that one of your social contacts is a certified WellPal are high. And they offer their help and advice without charging you.

WellPals will be able to answer your questions like:
- "My chest hurts; should I take an aspirin or a Tylenol?" Answer: Call 911 and go to the emergency department.
- "My blood pressure is 170/100. Shall I try my herbs, or do I need to seek medical attention?" Answer: Go to your doctor!
- "I have diabetes, and my blood sugar is well controlled. My cholesterol is normal, yet my doctor insists on me taking a statin. I'm afraid statin will destroy my liver. What should I do?" Answer: Diabetes is an artery disease. To protect your arteries, your LDL cholesterol level should be lower than "normal" because you are a diabetic and have very sensitive arteries. Statins (and other medications that lower LDL) reduce heart attacks and strokes. Take them!
- "Alzheimer's runs in my family. What can I do to reduce my risk?" Answer: Do what you need to do to avoid artery disease (healthy diet, adequate exercise and sleep, limited sitting time, control your blood pressure, LDL and blood sugar, avoid obesity) and avoid brain injuries. What is good for your arteries is also good for your brain!
- "My mom had diabetes; I sit all the time in front of a computer, and I have a big belly. But I am only 19 years old. I don't need to have my blood sugar checked, do I?" Answer: Of course you do. Your risk of developing diabetes is significant, in spite of your young age. There are now lots of children and adolescents with (type 2) diabetes, something that we did not see 40 years ago.

Why WellPals?

WellPals are the natural extension of community programs, like teaching CPR to non-professionals. The openness of the medical community to extending teaching medical skills, like CPR, to non-professionals, has been met by such a great success that need not be limited to CPR alone. What about teaching skills to willing and capable individuals about preventing diabetes and heart attacks?

Here are the reasons:
- As cardiac arrest is a true emergency, type 2 diabetes and artery disease are "an emergency in slow motion," according to the Secretary General of the United Nations.
- Diabetes and artery disease, after they silently destroy our arteries for some time, are themselves common causes of cardiac arrest.
- Diabetes and artery disease are much more common than cardiac arrest; a person who learns CPR may never actually perform it. On the other hand, a person who learns about belly fat, type 2 diabetes, high blood pressure, and abnormal cholesterol will have multiple, if not daily, opportunities to apply those skills.
- As obesity, diabetes, and artery disease are "upstream" conditions (predate) in regards to CPR, preventing them or getting individuals suffering from them to their primary care providers is a lifesaver (I can't tell you how many of these people absolutely refuse to see their healthcare providers).

Doesn't it make sense to act early enough, to educate and advise our fellow human beings and prevent cardiac arrest from happening in the first place? It's a fact that too many people trust the advice of their friends and loved ones on health matters. Wouldn't be great if your friend or loved one who offers an informal health advice has actually been trained and certified in obesity-diabetes-artery disease prevention?

Consider that, while only 8% of cardiac arrest victims who undergo CPR survive, so many more individuals are at high risk for cardiac arrest due to the obesity-related diseases, as:

- 10% of the population are diabetics
- One out of three adults have prediabetes
- One out of two adults has high blood pressure
- Cholesterol plaques are present in the heart arteries of two out of three seemingly healthy adults (especially men) as early as in their late twenties and early thirties
- Obesity, diabetes, heart disease, and stroke cost us almost one trillion USD per year, and costs continue to climb. These costs threaten not only the health of the diabetes and artery disease victims but also the welfare of our society.

How about YOU becoming a WellPal?

- You want to help.
  - You want to help so that yourself, your loved ones, your colleagues, and your fellow human beings avoid the perils of diabetes and artery disease.
- You want to make a difference in our society.
  - People volunteer to work in hospitals helping the sick. Isn't it equally important to help your friends and family from becoming sick?
- You want to develop new skills and acquire new knowledge.
- You may be looking to build your resume or find employment.
  - This type of knowledge will help you. Employers want to keep their employees healthy and happy and, having knowledgeable people like you, can make a difference in their team.
- You want to get involved in your community and get to know people around you.
- You are looking for a purpose or being inspired by a good cause.
  - The obesity-diabetes-artery disease epidemic concerns us all and is a threat to our society and our economy.

Chapter 7 Questions

1. How can school curriculum help raise awareness about obesity and diabetes among children?

2. What object's removal from the classroom will help young kids increase the amount of physical activities they complete during school?

3. What type of food is the most dangerous for the health of kids, adolescents, and young, middle aged, and elderly adults?

4. Mention one great success story of public health in the United States. How long did it take to see these spectacular achievements?

5. Why do people trust their friends' advice in health matters?

6. Mention four behaviors/actions that show that a middle-aged individual takes responsibility for his/her health.

7. Is it possible for an intelligent and well-motivated individual to learn enough details about preventive medicine so that he or she can become a credible source of advice for their loved ones and social contacts? Explain.

8. Why are modern hospitals, the way they currently operate, not effective agents of disease prevention in the community?

9. Who is most likely to defeat the obesity-diabetes-artery disease epidemic?

10. Who are the "**WellPals**," and how can they help in the fight against the obesity-diabetes-artery disease epidemic?

11. What lessons can we learn from the ways Aristotle was teaching his students in the Peripatetic School of Aristotle?

12. What lessons does the dissemination of CPR training in the community hold for the fight against the obesity-diabetes-artery disease epidemic?

13. Why is performing a lot of physical activities during work the only way for the working American to achieve the requirements for healthy living in regards to physical activities and exercise?

Chapter 8

EPILOGUE

Aging and retirement in the time of obesity and diabetes

"I'm not telling you it's going to be easy—I'm telling you it's going to be worth it"
—Art Williams

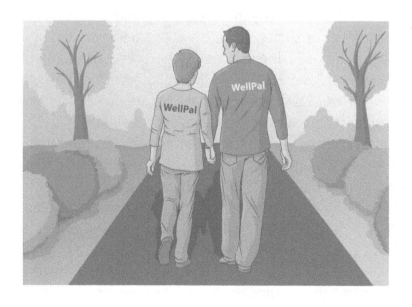

Every day we are different people, especially on the inside: our beta cells are different, the linings of our arteries are different, our cholesterol plaques are different. While the face we look at the mirror remains, more or less, the same face it was yesterday, inside us there is a different reality. Billions of new cells are "born" to replace cells that got old and died. Every day we lose some muscle, some pancreas beta cells, some kidney filtration units. "Senescence" is the word science uses to describe the millions of changes that happen, day after day, as we get older. And, of course, our chromosomes' telomeres, the time clocks of our life, get shorter and shorter.

So, how do we fare as we get older in a world deeply affected by obesity, diabetes, and artery disease? What are the things we should or can do as we are getting older? What are the new realities we face every day as time piles up on us? What does "old" really mean? And what do we want to leave behind for the next generation?

Younger people may be tempted to think that once our fifties or sixties are gone, life doesn't have any more exciting things to offer. But if you ask those in their fifties or sixties, you are likely to get a very different picture:

- "Over-sixties see themselves in the prime of life," wrote Sarah Womack, in June 2004 in a UK publication (*The Telegraph*). "A fifth of those over 75 still believe that they are middle-aged, and a third consider themselves very attractive for their age."
- A study by the Pew Research Center in 2013 found that only 21% of Americans aged 65 to 74 say that they feel old. Even among people over 75, only 35% call themselves old. In another study, Harvard University researchers surveyed Americans aged between 55 and 74 and found that the average person in this age group feels 12 years younger than their age.

And while it is true that old age comes with less energy, slower metabolism, thinner hair, more wrinkles, fewer muscles, and fewer functioning pancreas beta cells, weaker bones, higher blood pressure, and stiffer arteries and heart muscle, it also comes with more experience, more available time for ourselves and our loved ones, fewer direct responsibilities, and more benevolence and humility. It may sound as an oxymoron, but it is only during the latter part of our lives that, in spite of physical weaknesses and limitations, we are as strong as it takes to do or say certain things that we could not possibly do or say during our heydays (like anything that would have jeopardized our job or offended our boss, for example). And, thanks to better sanitation conditions, more widespread awareness about wellness, and improved medical care, opportunities to do the things we always wanted to but couldn't abound as the "elderly"—those 65 years or older—is the fastest growing segment in our society.

Here is what CDC has to say: "Older Americans can expect to live longer than ever before. Under existing conditions, women who live to age 65 can expect to live about 19 years longer, men about 16 years longer."

What is "old age," and what can you expect from it?

What scientists and institutions consider as "old age" varies significantly. Using "chronological age" (the number of years a person has lived), the range starts at 60 and ends at 85-plus. For example:
- The United Nations consider any age above 60 years as "old age."
- Most Western countries set the age for retirement at 60–65.
- In order to qualify for full Social Security benefits, you must be at least 67 years old.
- Some scientists divide old age into several groups with the "old-old" defined as 85-plus.

Biological age, on the other hand, has to do with how quickly (or slowly) or how well (or badly) we age (our body, our arteries and other organs, and our cells). Biological age has to do not only with our chronological age but also with our genes and lifestyle. We have all met (and been surprised by) people who look younger (or older) and perform better (or worse) than their chronological age. Taking how well people function into "old age," sociologists Paul Higgs and Chris Gilleard divide "old age" into two parts:
- "**third age**" as "the period in life of active retirement, following middle age" and
- "**fourth age**" as the period of "inactive, unhealthy, unproductive, and ultimately unsuccessful ageing."

(in *Rethinking Old Age: Theorizing the Fourth Age*, Palgrave Macmillan, 2015). In other words, getting older or retiring from work does not mean that our life has ended, as our "third age" can be a very productive one.

The effect of lifestyle on our health during old age

While even the healthiest of lifestyles will not make us immortal, it will, nevertheless, significantly increase not only our lifespan (how many years we live) but, most importantly, our healthspan (how many years we live in good health). In this way, healthy lifestyle earlier in life will shorten the suffering, incapacitation, and loss of autonomy and dignity. Increases in longevity close to 15 years along with less pain, suffering, and disability, fewer surgeries, and an improved capacity to function can be realized when we stick to a healthy lifestyle, especially if we start early in life. And what helps prevent obesity, diabetes, and artery disease also helps prevent Alzheimer's, cancer, depression, falls, and the need to go to the nursing home.

According to CDC, "Whether the added years at the end of the life cycle are healthy, enjoyable, and productive depends, in part, upon **preventing and controlling a number of chronic diseases and conditions.**" In other words, if you have not taken care of your body earlier in life, old age is likely to bring pain, incapacitation, and suffering, frequently in the form of diabetes, arthritis, heart attacks, heart failure, atrial fibrillation, stroke, cancer, emphysema, or Alzheimer's. So, have you done your homework during your earlier years? Have you invested in your health? **How much have you saved for your health in retirement?**

As we have seen in Chapter 5, the key elements of a healthy lifestyle are:
- Not smoking
- Staying thin
- Moving around for a few hours every day
- Eating healthy (lots of fruits and vegetables, no added sugars, few animal fats, and small quantities of the good fats)
- Respecting the day/night cycle and getting at least seven hours of sleep per night
- Avoiding extreme and unnatural stress and too many worries
- Restricting the use of medications like NSAIDs and opioids

- Keeping a rich and vibrant social life (this is especially true as we grow older)

This lifestyle will help you reach anywhere from your late seventies to your nineties (depending on your genes and a little bit of luck) and in good shape so you can work or play and enjoy grandkids or travelling, as:

- Aerobic, strengthening, and balance exercises, if consistently practiced earlier in life, have probably given you a strong, muscular body with less osteoporosis, better mobility, and independence (no falls!).
- Reducing your salt intake reduces the chances you develop high blood pressure, heart failure, or suffer a stroke.
- Avoiding obesity reduces the chances of becoming diabetic or developing heart attacks, stroke, heart failure, and knee arthritis.
- Not smoking will make it less likely that you develop emphysema, lung or throat cancer, heart attacks, stroke, and aneurysms.
- Avoiding alcohol abuse reduces the chances of developing liver failure, heart failure, atrial fibrillation (a stroke-prone type of irregular heart rhythm), or stroke.
- A blood pressure that has been maintained in the normal range (no more than 140/90 mmHg for most of us, controlled through a healthy lifestyle or medications, if necessary) will significantly reduce the chances of stroke, heart attack, heart failure, and atrial fibrillation.

The effect of a healthy lifestyle on brain health is particularly important, as dementia can render life meaningless for the individual and a heavy burden for loved ones and society.

We only live once, so reaching your eighties or nineties in good shape makes the human experience richer, as you are able to "watch" the entire play in the theater of life: youth, middle and older age, work and retirement, strength and vulnerability, enthusiasm and experience, parents and children, grandparents and grandkids, successes and failures, arrogance and humility, hurting or being hurt and, hopefully, benevolence and forgiveness.

The many challenges of retirement

It is true that most people do not like their jobs. According to a Gallup's 142-country study on the *State of the Global Workplace* in 2013, about 70 percent of US and Canada workers are not actively engaged in their job (read: they don't like their job), with all other countries in the study ranking even lower. With so few of us liking our jobs, it is no wonder that we look up to retirement to liberate us from the scourge of daily labor. In reality, however, retirement is a mixed blessing, especially for those who did not plan carefully ahead of retirement time. It is true that retirement delivers us from our boss and the alarm clock and opens up vast amounts of free time, but it also challenges us:

- Financially, as it reduces our income, so, in case we didn't save enough for retirement, we may have to forgo the lifestyle that we were used to (a comfortable home, two cars, or travelling abroad).
- Socially, as it separates us from colleagues and decade-old friends.
- Emotionally, as it may make us feel we are no longer productive elements of the society and we no longer have a purpose in life. These feelings of unworthiness may bring on depression, which while serious, may be difficult to diagnose.

As **retirement coincides with aging**, it shakes us to the core and causes a huge **identity crisis,** as big as the one during adolescence but in the reverse direction. During this "reverse adolescence":

- We change physically. We develop wrinkles, white hair, brittle bones, and arthritis, and we lose muscle.
- We change functionally. Energy is down, balance becomes more difficult, gait may become unsteady, joints hurt and become stiff, and we are no longer capable of doing the things we used to.
- Our sex drive declines, and we are no longer as attractive as we used to be.
- Our social environment changes drastically. We may distance ourselves from former co-workers and decades-old friends, and we may lose loved ones to sickness or death. Our kids see us differently, as both our income and physical capacities are down and we can no longer be the solid rock they once could lean on.

- We change emotionally. Loss of strength and purpose along with loneliness frequently lead to anxiety or depression and even alcohol, opioid, and sedative abuse.
- We lose independence. We may become more dependent on family members and under terms that are neither of our choice nor of our liking. At some point, the specter of nursing home may become a necessity.
- Health problems develop: high blood pressure, arthritis, diabetes, cancer, atrial fibrillation, heart failure, heart attacks, and strokes. We may find ourselves taking a large number of pills (that while helping our original condition also have side effects). We frequently need to visit multiple doctors (primary care and specialists), each one looking at only the part of our body they're supposed to treat with competing goals among them. Our primary care and orthopedic doctor may recommend daily ibuprofen for our knee arthritis, but our kidney doctor and cardiologist warn us against these medications—NSAIDs—since, when taken daily they can shut down our kidneys and hearts, leading to dialysis, heart attacks, or heart failure. Our ever-increasing copays and deductibles hurt our frequently tight budget. While most medications used are generics and are supposed to be inexpensive, their price in the US is significantly higher than it is in most European countries, even as their manufacturer is the same. According to a Bloomberg report in December 2015 by Robert Langreth et al, "Even after an estimated discount of 60 percent, AstraZeneca still charges more than twice as much in the U.S. for Crestor, a cholesterol pill, compared to Germany, and in other countries the price is even lower, according to the analysis of IHS data."

So, **plan your retirement** well ahead of time, with focus on:
- **Sustainable finances**, with expenses commensurate to income, keeping in mind that Social Security may not be there for future generations.
- A **structured schedule** through daily physical activities, part-time employment, volunteering, learning something new, reading books, travelling as much as your budget and health allow; fill your daily life with physical and mental challenges.

- Maintaining a **rich social life**: rekindle old friendships and make new ones, opting for some friends younger than you.
- Reaching older life **as healthy as possible:** strong, muscular, and without belly fat, with good balance and functionality, sharp both in the physical and mental departments.
- **Self-monitoring your health regularly**: make it a habit. As soon as you wake up, empty your bladder and then weigh yourself wearing only your underwear; then, go back to your bed, rest for five minutes, and take your blood pressure and pulse rate. If your weight or blood pressure fluctuates little from day to day, you may monitor these once or twice a week. Monitor the number of your daily steps and aim at at least 15,000 steps a day through moderate-pace walking. Monitor your waist circumference once a week.
- **Knowing what medicines you take** and for what reason: every time you visit your doctor, bring the actual medication bottles with you. Include supplements and over-the-counter medications.
- **Knowing your "numbers"**: your blood pressure, blood sugar, A1c, and LDL cholesterol are musts. Hemoglobin, creatinine, triglycerides, and HDL cholesterol are also important.
- **Keeping your own medical file** consisting of your hospital admissions, medical and surgical procedures, and results of outpatient testing. Due to regulations (HIPAA, "data privacy and security provisions for safeguarding medical information") and the fact that many hospitals and outpatient centers destroy records that are older than 10 years, it is difficult for your current health care providers to obtain your previous health records. Every time you have a test done, ask for a copy of the report; remember that such reports are written in medical terminology and, unless your provider explains the key points, going over them is likely to raise more questions than answers.
- A **productive partnership with your doctor**, most importantly your primary care provider, so that you are kept up to date with screening tests (like colonoscopies and mammograms) and immunizations (like flu shots, pneumococcal and herpes zoster vaccines) and reporting any new symptoms so that disease can be diagnosed earlier and treated more effectively.

The price of neglect

Not planning ahead for your retirement, not keeping a structured daily schedule, and neglecting your health comes at a price. According to the Health and Retirement Study (a large, state of the art, ongoing US study of aging, health, retirement, disability, and family support), there was an increase of 40% in heart attacks and stroke during the first year of retirement, as compared to those who keep working.

Sitting in front of a TV, a computer screen, or in a couch the entire day sets you up for:
- Obesity and diabetes
- Depression
- Alzheimer's
- Heart disease and stroke

How to avoid all these:
- Limit the time you spend sitting to no more than six hours a day.
- Stay physically and socially active; go out with friends.
- Walk and lift light weights every day.
- Stimulate your brain by reading, studying, playing musical instruments, and learning something new every day.
- Volunteer.
- Have a part time job.

The shockwaves produced by the retirement of baby boomers

The baby boomers, 76 million people born during the "baby boom" years, from 1946 to 1964, after an unsuccessful attempt at early retirement that was shuttered by the Great Recession of 2007, are now finally retiring. The massive retirement of skilled workers that defined an epoch is likely to send shockwaves to the:
- Labor market
- Health care and Medicare
- Social Security

Almost 4 million people a year will turn from taxpayers to Social Security and Medicare beneficiaries. The cost of Social Security will rise faster than tax income because the population over age 65 will grow faster than the working-age population. On top of the talent, productivity, and tax money lost, baby boomers have their own unique health problems. While they did not smoke as much as their predecessors, the "silent generation," according to CDC, retiring baby boomers are expected to have more diabetes (one in five persons) and more high blood pressure (one in two). As healthcare costs for diabetics are more than double the costs for non-diabetics, baby boomers' retirement will be an expensive stress test for Medicare. And in spite their increased diabetes and obesity rates, baby boomers are expected to live longer than previous generations, drawing more Social Security benefits and incurring even more Medicare costs.

In the 2014 edition of the *Annual Report of the Board of Trustees of the Federal Old-Age and Survivors Insurance and Federal Disability Insurance Trust Funds*, "**reserves are projected to peak around 2020 and to be depleted around 2033** if no changes are made to the tax or benefit provisions before then."

Quality versus quantity of life

As we succeed in extending life expectancy, CDC, along with most of us, asks this all-important question: "What will these added years bring? Will they be spent in active, productive, fulfilling endeavors, or will they be overshadowed by declining health, loss of memory, and lingering illness? How valuable is a longer life if we simply increase the time we spend functionally limited by such debilitating ailments as heart disease, osteoporosis, or Alzheimer's disease?"

Alzheimer's: a serious but potentially preventable disease of the elderly

Death from Alzheimer's disease ranks fifth among causes of death in individuals aged 65 and over in the US. According to Alzheimer Society Canada, healthy lifestyle can significantly reduce the risk of one of the most feared diseases that affects the elderly: Alzheimer's disease and other dementias. These important but modifiable risk factors account for almost half of the cases of dementia:

- Diabetes
- High blood pressure
- Obesity
- Smoking
- Depression
- Cognitive inactivity or low education
- Physical inactivity

The similarities between what prevents artery disease and dementia are striking; those healthy habits that help prevent heart attacks and stroke also reduce significantly the risk of dementia. So, both in terms of becoming an epidemic over the last 25 years and in terms of their risk profile, Alzheimer's and other types of dementia parallel the obesity-diabetes-artery disease epidemic.

This information appears on the Alzheimer's Organization website:

"The Mayo clinic advocates maintaining an active lifestyle as one of the most effective ways to prevent the onset of Alzheimer's or dementia. This may include attending social gatherings, playing sports, or engaging in mentally-challenging activities (puzzles, games, reading).

Dr Glenn Smith, a neuropsychologist with the Mayo Clinic specializing in Alzheimer's, recommends:

- Avoid smoking, as smoking has shown to increase the chance of developing Alzheimer's by 80 percent.
- Eat a balanced diet rich in vegetables, fruits, and lean protein, particularly protein sources containing omega-3 fatty acids.
- Be physically active; aim for going for a walk each day, but at least a minimum of three times a week.
- Be socially active; spend time with your friends or family at least once a week. Social activity is some of the best mental stimulation.
- Take care of your mental health.
- Use thinking (cognitive) skills, such as memory skills.

And he continues: "One of the best ways to engage in these activities is to become active in your community. Even attending an event once a week may be enough to prevent the onset of dementia or Alzheimer's."

Getting enough sleep, using vitamins B complex (B3, B6, B12, and folic acid), D, and E, taking time to relax and destress, and reducing alcohol intake also appear on the Alzheimer's Organization's recommendations.

Death from natural causes

Death is the natural end of our life cycle and, as we mentioned earlier, even the most perfect lifestyle and best genes cannot prevent it. As a result, there is the notion of "death due to natural causes." What does it mean? Well, there is no exact meaning other than excluding death due to accidents, homicide, or suicide. "Peaceful" is one word that comes to mind when we mention "natural" death. And a peaceful death at an old age, without suffering, at our own home, and surrounded by loved ones is both a blessing and a privilege. I challenge you to consider under what conditions so many fellow human beings have died over the centuries of history or are nowadays dying in hospital ICUs.

"Natural" death may be sudden or following a more or less prolonged illness. Sudden death at an "older" age (e.g., in our eighties) is usually considered "natural," even if the precise cause is unknown, although there is always some specific cause of death. Was it a heart attack, a stroke, or a clot in the lungs? In reality, there is always something pathological that kills us; we do not die of "natural" death when everything is "normal." Frequent causes of "natural death" among older people include killer blood clots (stroke, heart attack, or a large clot in the lungs), widespread cancer, infections (pneumonia), or a brain that lost too many cells and cell connections due to Alzheimer's or Parkinson's disease. On the contrary, a sudden death in a younger person without a diagnosed previous illness is not considered "natural death," and a coroner may require an autopsy to be performed to determine the cause of death.

The distinction among sudden death in older versus younger people undermines an important feature of our biology as we age: **death in the**

old-old (let's say 85+) is a built-in feature of the human body, independent of how great our previous lifestyle has been or how wonderful are genes are. Nature has provided our bodies with internal executable programs that reside in our genes and, as we age, make us much more likely to die of a clot, an uncontrolled cancer, or loss of nerve cells and mishandling of their proteins. And this is inherent in human species and above and beyond wear and tear of our organs. The human body is designed from the beginning of our life to last no more than a century (more or less); the shortening telomeres in our chromosomes are a reflection (although not necessarily the cause) of our programmed death at an old-old age. This is something that, with our current level of technology, we cannot change, not even with a perfect lifestyle. What a healthy lifestyle may provide us, though, as the end approaches, is that we retain our ability to function (with only simple support, like a cane, eyeglasses, or hearing aids) to the very end and, thus, shorten the time of incapacitation, suffering, or dementia.

Here are two important comments by human aging scientists:
- Alex Smith, an assistant professor of medicine at the University of California in San Francisco in 2013 states that: "natural death is something more like a peaceful death, free from invasive medical interventions." (interventions like ventilators, CPR, and artificial hearts in ICU)
- A sudden death not preceded by a prolonged period of pain, suffering incapacitation, and being a burden to our family in our late eighties seems, beyond being "natural," the best way to go for most of us. And a previously healthy lifestyle, while unable to make us immortal, can "compress" the period of disability to the absolute minimum, according to a study published on the September 2017 issue of the *Journal of the American Geriatrics Society* by M. Jacob, LM Yee et al. These researchers reported that "the effects of healthy lifestyle factors on the proportion of future life lived free of disability indicate that the disabled period (at the end of life) can be compressed, given the right combination of these (healthy lifestyle) factors." So, eating right, exercising, sleeping well, avoiding prolonged sitting, being a non-smoker, avoiding abuse alcohol or drugs, and maintaining a rich social life, will not only help us live

longer and healthier but will also shorten the last and most dreaded part of life, the "fourth age" of suffering and incapacitation, helping us maintain good functionality, independence, and freedom from pain and medical procedures and allowing us to keep pour dignity to almost the very end. Isn't this a worthy goal for you?

What do we want your legacy to be?

As you are wrapping up your life, what do you want your legacy to be? How and what do you want to be remembered for? Beyond your estate, what do you want to leave for your children and grandchildren, for the next generation? Perhaps you want to leave some piece of advice for your kids or grandkids, a few written pages with your life's highlights or particular experiences, things you did and should have not done or things you did not do and regretted for not doing. You may want to write a book with your memoirs. As you reach an older age, you become more free in the sense that you can open up about things you did not want to explicitly discuss when you were younger. You no longer have to be "politically correct." There is no boss to insult, no job to be afraid of losing; you are done with most of your direct responsibilities to your kids and to society. Speak up! Say it now! Is there anything you have been holding back all these years? Any particular feelings about people around you, your spouse, your kids, your friends, your parents, your bosses, politicians, the society in general, the arts, the direction this world is moving to? Being healthy, bright, and energetic enough during your later years in life can give you this unique opportunity to discuss uncomfortable truths. Opening up this way can be so liberating; it may lift a huge burden off of you and set you free. It will add to the "human experience," what this life meant to you, looking at it from this vantage point unfettered by biases and responsibilities that could have prevented you from being that open in previous years.

And if you experienced the benefits of a healthy lifestyle and lived a longer, more vibrant, more optimistic, and happier life, isn't it worth it to pass it down to your kids and grandkids? Why not help the cause of fighting against the obesity-diabetes-artery disease epidemic?

If you think that changing our schools, the workplace, and ourselves is too difficult or even impossible, then think of the alternative: as far as this planet is concerned, the human race does not necessarily need to survive another century, let alone another millenium.

Chapter 8 Questions

1. Mention four benefits of retirement.

2. What are the health risks associated with retirement?

3. Is retirement a stress-free period? If so, why? If not, why not?

4. Mention six behaviors that reduce the risk of Alzheimer's and other forms of dementia

5. Does obesity or diabetes increase the risk of dementia?

6. What do sociologists Paul Higgs and Chris Gilleard mean by "3rd" and "4th" age?

7. Are the baby boomers financially prepared for retirement?

8. What are the socioeconomic consequences of the retirement of baby boomers?

9. Ever since you retired, you have been watching TV for eight hours a day. What's wrong with that?

References

https://www.cdc.gov/media/releases/2017/p0718-diabetes-report.html

http://www.who.int/diabetes/country-profiles/mex_en.pdf?ua=1

https://www.ncbi.nlm.nih.gov/pubmed/25241351

https://www.cdc.gov/obesity/data/adult.html

https://www.nhlbi.nih.gov/sites/default/files/media/docs/obesity-evidence-review.pdf

Managing Overweight and Obesity in Adults. Systematic Evidence Review From the Obesity Expert Panel, 2013, U.S. Department of Health and Human Services, National Institutes of Health, National Heart, Lung and Blood Institute

Wing RR1 et al; Look AHEAD Research Group.Benefits of modest weight loss in improving cardiovascular risk factors in overweight and obese individuals with type 2 diabetes. Diabetes Care. 2011;34(7):1481-6.

Walker KZ1, O'Dea K, Gomez M, Girgis S, Colagiuri R.Diet and exercise in the prevention of Diabetes. J Hum Nutr Diet. 2010;23(4):344-52.

Action for Health in Diabetes (Look AHEAD) Trial,
Baseline evaluation of selected nutrients and food group intake
Mara Z. Vitolins, DrPH, MPH, RD, et al, and Look AHEAD Research Group,
J Am Diet Assoc. 2009 Aug; 109(8): 1367–1375.

The Future Financial Status of the Social Security Program
by Stephen C. Goss, Social Security Bulletin, Vol. 70, No. 3, 2010

https://www.heritage.org/health-care-reform/report/medicares-next-50-years-preserving-the-prog ram-future-retirees

Jose Miguel Baena-Díez et al.on behalf of the FRESCO Investigators: Risk of Cause-Specific
Death in Individuals With Diabetes: A Competing Risks Analysis
Diabetes Care 2016 Nov; 39(11): 1987-1995

Despres JP, Lemieux I. Abdominal obesity and metabolic syndrome. Nature 2006;444:881-7. 10.1038/nature05488

https://www.cdc.gov/obesity/adult/causes.html

https://www.mayoclinic.org/diseases-conditions/obesity/diagnosis-treatment/drc-20375749

The Epidemiology of Obesity: A Big Picture Adela Hruby, PhD, MPH and Frank B. Hu, MD, PhD, MPH
Pharmacoeconomics. 2015 Jul; 33(7): 673–689.

Age-Related Impairment of Pancreatic Beta-Cell Function: Pathophysiological and Cellular Mechanisms
Vincenzo De Tata1,*
Front Endocrinol (Lausanne). 2014; 5: 138.

https://www.bloomberg.com/news/articles/2017-07-10/working-past-70-americans-can-t-seem-t o-retire

https://www.alz.org/national/documents/latino_brochure_diabetes.pdf

Relationship between Added Sugars Consumption and Chronic Disease Risk Factors: Current Understanding
James M. Rippe and Theodore J. Angelopoulos
Nutrients. 2016 Nov; 8(11): 697.

https://www.hhs.gov/about/strategic-plan/introduction/index.html

https://www.cdc.gov

https://www.nih.gov/about-nih/who-we-are

https://www.cms.gov

https://www.cdc.gov/nchs/nvss/vsrr/mortality.htm

Projecting the Future Diabetes Population Size and Related Costs for the U.S. Elbert S. Huang, MD, MPH, Anirban Basu, PHD, Michael O'Grady, PHD, and James C. Capretta, MA
Diabetes Care. 2009 Dec; 32(12): 2225–2229

http://www.who.int/bulletin/mission_statement/en

Abdobesity: The Belly Fat That Kills by AJ Pothoulakis and GY Demosthenous

https://news.heart.org/cpr-skills-low-among-older-adults

https://www.aafp.org/fpm/2004/0600/p68.html

http://www.newsweek.com/healthy-habits-could-boost-life-expectancy-15-years-harvard-study-9 05553

https://www.cdc.gov/tobacco/campaign/tips/resources/data/cigarette-smoking-in-united-states.ht ml

https://asmbs.org/patients

https://www.theguardian.com/commentisfree/2014/jul/14/bariatric-surgery-no-cure-all-obesity

http://www.apa.org/helpcenter/understanding-chronic-stress.aspx

Atherothrombosis: A widespread disease with unpredictable and life-threatening consequences Juan F Viles-Gonzalez Valentin Fuster Juan J Badimon
European Heart Journal, Volume 25, Issue 14, 1 July 2004, Pages 1197–1207

https://en.wikipedia.org/wiki/Cell_(biology)

https://www.mayoclinic.org/diseases-conditions/nonalcoholic-fatty-liver-disease/symptoms-caus es/syc-20354567

http://www.joslin.org/info/what_is_insulin_resistance.html

Ectopic and Visceral Fat Deposition in Lean and Obese Patients With Type 2 Diabetes Eylem Levelt, MBBS, DPhil, et al.
J Am Coll Cardiol. 2016 Jul 5; 68(1): 53–63.

Coutinho T, Goel K, Corrêa de Sa´ D, et al. Central obesity and survival in subjects with coronary artery disease: a systematic review of the published data and collaborative analysis with individual subject data. J Am Coll Cardiol 2011;57:1877– 86.

PATHOPHYSIOLOGY AND TREATMENT OF TYPE 2 DIABETES: PERSPECTIVES ON THE PAST, PRESENT AND FUTURE
Steven E. Kahn, M.B., Ch.B., Mark E. Cooper, M.B., B.S, Ph.D., and Stefano Del Prato, M.D. Lancet. 2014 Mar 22; 383(9922): 1068–1083.

https://www.diabetes.co.uk/difference-between-type1-and-type2-diabetes.html

ABC of hypertension:The pathophysiology of hypertension
Gareth Beevers, Gregory Y H Lip, and Eoin O'Brien
BMJ. 2001 Apr 14; 322(7291): 912–916.

https://www.uspharmacist.com/article/cardiometabolic-syndrome-a-global-health-issue

Modern Biological Theories of Aging Kunlin Jin
Aging Dis. 2010 Oct; 1(2): 72–74.

http://www.biology-pages.info/C/Cholesterol.html

Sleep Duration and Cardiovascular Disease Risk: Epidemiologic and Experimental Evidence Naima Covassin, PhD and Prachi singh, PhD
Sleep Med Clin. 2016 Mar; 11(1): 81–89.

Sleep duration predicts cardiovascular outcomes: a systematic review and meta-analysis of prospective studies
Francesco P. Cappuccio Daniel Cooper Lanfranco D'Elia Pasquale Strazzullo Michelle A. Miller European Heart Journal, Volume 32, Issue 12, 1 June 2011, Pages 1484–1492

J.F. PAGEL, MD, MS, Rocky Mountain Sleep Disorders Center, Pueblo, Colorado Am Fam Physician. 2009 Mar 1;79(5):391-396.

https://www.niddk.nih.gov/health-information/diabetes/overview/tests-diagnosis/a1c-test

https://en.wikipedia.org/wiki/Articular_cartilage_damage

Microvascular and Macrovascular Complications of Diabetes Michael J. Fowler, MD
Clinical Diabetes 2008 Apr; 26(2): 77-82.

AGING AND MUSCLE MORPHOLOGY: LINKING AGE-RELATED CHANGES IN SKELETAL MUSCLE MASS AND COMPOSITION WITH METABOLISM AND DISEASE
I. JANSSEN, R. ROSS
The Journal of Nutrition, Health & Aging© Volume 9, Number 6, 2005

Lifestyle, social factors, and survival after age 75: population based study Debora Rizzuto, PhD student, Nicola Orsini, associate professor, Chengxuan Qiu, associate professor, Hui-Xin Wang, senior researcher, Laura Fratiglioni, professor
BMJ 2012; 345

Will All Americans Become Overweight or Obese? Estimating the Progression and Cost of the US Obesity Epidemic
Youfa Wang, May A. Beydoun, Lan Liang, Benjamin Caballero and Shiriki K. Kumanyika Obesity (2008) 16, 2323–2330.

Trends in Cardiovascular Health Metrics and Associations With All-Cause and CVD Mortality Among US Adults

Quanhe Yang, PhD; Mary E. Cogswell, DrPH; W. Dana Flanders, MD, ScD; et al Yuling Hong, MD, PhD; Zefeng Zhang, MD, PhD; Fleetwood Loustalot, FNP, PhD; Cathleen Gillespie, MS; Robert Merritt, BA, MA; Frank B. Hu, MD, PhD
JAMA. 2012;307(12):1273-1283. doi:10.1001/jama.2012.339

https://www.cdc.gov/nchs/fastats/leading-causes-of-death.htm

Long working hours and risk of coronary heart disease and stroke: a systematic review and meta-analysis of published and unpublished data for 603 838 individuals
Prof Mika Kivimäki, PhD et al., The Lancet, Volume 386, No. 10005, p1739–1746, 31 October 2015

Cardiovascular safety of non-steroidal anti-inflammatory drugs: network meta-analysis Sven Trelle, senior research fellow et al.
BMJ 2011; 342:c7086

Association of Coffee Drinking with Total and Cause-Specific Mortality
Neal D. Freedman, Ph.D., Yikyung Park, Sc.D., Christian C. Abnet, Ph.D., Albert R. Hollenbeck, Ph.D., and Rashmi Sinha, Ph.D.
N Engl J Med 2012; 366:1891-1904

https://www.samhsa.gov

https://www.niaaa.nih.gov/alcohol-health/alcohols-effects-body

https://www.drugabuse.gov/publications/drugfacts/marijuana

https://www.drugabuse.gov/publications/research-reports/cocaine/what-are-short-term-effects-c ocaine-use

https://www.drugabuse.gov/publications/research-reports/heroin/what-are-immediate-short-term-effects-heroin-use

https://adf.org.au/drug-facts/heroin/

https://medlineplus.gov/methamphetamine.html

https://www.fda.gov/Food/DietarySupplements

https://www.cdc.gov/vaccines/schedules/index.html

https://www.cancer.org/healthy/find-cancer-early/cancer-screening-guidelines/american-cancer-society-guidelines-for-the-early-detection-of-cancer.html

https://www.washingtonpost.com/news/wonk/wp/2015/06/02/medical-researchers-have-figured-out-how-much-time-is-okay-to-spend-sitting-each-day/?noredirect=on&utm_term=.286f84adecd a

Am J Prev Med. 2011 Aug;41(2):178-88. doi: 10.1016/j.amepre.2011.05.002.
Sedentary behavior and dietary intake in children, adolescents, and adults. A systematic review. Pearson N1, Biddle SJ.

https://www.cdc.gov/healthliteracy/education-support/schools.html

https://cpr.heart.org/AHAECC/CPRAndECC/UCM_473161_CPR-and-ECC.jsp

https://www.ncvo.org.uk/ncvo-volunteering/why-volunteer

https://en.wikipedia.org/wiki/Peripatetic_school

https://www.thewalkingclassroom.org/

https://www.alz.org/documents_custom/2017-facts-and-figures.pdf

https://www.thediabetescouncil.com/can-you-work-if-you-have-diabetes/

CPSIA information can be obtained
at www.ICGtesting.com
Printed in the USA
FSHW020855081118
53467FS

9 781946 697998